# Guide to Targeted Therapies:
# EGFR Mutations in NSCLC

Federico Cappuzzo
Director, Medical Oncology Department
Istituto Toscano Tumori-Ospedale Civile di Livorno
Livorno, Italy

# Guide to Targeted Therapies: EGFR Mutations in NSCLC

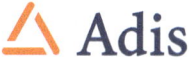

ISBN 978-3-319-03058-6   ISBN 978-3-319-03059-3 (eBook)
DOI 10.1007/978-3-319-03059-3
Springer Cham Heidelberg New York Dordrecht London

Printed on acid-free paper

Springer is part of Springer Science+Business Media (www.springer.com)

Project editor: Tess Salazar
Production: Patty Goldstein

# Contents

# Contents

# Author biography

**Federico Cappuzzo, MD,** has been the Director of the medical oncology department at the Istituto Toscano Tumori-Ospedale Civile-Livorno in Livorno, Italy since January 2010. In November 1992, he graduated, summa cum laude, in medicine and surgery at the Palermo University. In November 1996, he gained a degree, summa cum laude, in medical oncology at Milan University, followed by the European Society for Medical Oncology (ESMO) certification in medical oncology in 1997. From 1997 to 1999, he was recipient of an ESMO Fellowship on Gene Therapy of Lung Cancer at Institut Gustave Roussy in Villejuif (Paris). He then was an attending physician at the thoracic oncology unit at the Medical University of South Carolina in Charleston from April 2000 to September 2000. For six years, from November 2000 to 2006, he was an assistant professor at Ospedale Bellaria in Bologna. From November 2006 to January 2010, Dr Cappuzzo was an assistant professor in medical oncology at Istituto Clinico Humanitas IRCCS in Rozzano (Milan), and from January 2004 to November 2004 he was a visiting associate professor in medical oncology at University of Colorado in Denver.

Dr Cappuzzo is a member of the Italian Association in Medical Oncology (AIOM), ESMO, American Society Clinical Oncology (ASCO), International Association for the Study of Lung Cancer (IASCL), and since 2006 has been a member of the editorial board of *Lung Cancer*. In 2006 and 2009, he received research grants from the Italian Association for Cancer Research (AIRC) on targeted therapies in lung cancer and is the author of more than 130 papers in peer-review journals, mainly in translational research in lung cancer.

# Abbreviations

| | |
|---|---|
| **ALK** | anaplastic lymphoma kinase |
| **ARMS** | Amplification Refractory Mutation System |
| **ATP** | adenosine triphosphate |
| **CCP** | cationic conjugated polymer |
| **CTC** | circulating tumor cells |
| **dHPLC** | denaturing high-performance liquid chromatography |
| **EBUS** | endobronchial ultrasound |
| **EGFR** | epidermal growth factor receptor |
| **EGF** | epidermal growth factor |
| **EUS** | esophageal ultrasound |
| **FDA** | US Food and Drug Administration |
| **FFPE** | formalin-fixed paraffin-embedded |
| **FISH** | fluorescence in situ hybridization |
| **FNA** | fine-needle aspirate |
| **FRET** | fluorescence resonance energy transfer |
| **IgG** | immunoglobulin G |
| **IHC** | immunohistochemistry |
| **HER** | human epidermal growth factor receptor |
| **HR** | hazard ratio |
| **HRMA** | high-resolution melting analysis |
| **LNA** | locked nucleic acid |
| **MAPK** | mitogen-activated protein kinase |
| **Mig6** | mitogen-inducible gene 6 (also known as ralt, ERRFI1, or Gene 33) |
| **NSCLC** | non-small cell lung cancer |
| **PI3k** | phosphatidylinositol 3'-kinase |
| **PCR** | polymerase chain reaction |
| **PNA** | peptide nucleic acid |
| **ptDNA** | plasma tumor DNA |
| **SmartAMP** | Smart Amplification Process |
| **TGFa** | transforming growth factor alpha |

| TKI | tyrosine kinase inhibitors |
| TTP | time to progression |
| WT | wild type |

# Preface

Non-small cell lung cancer (NSCLC) tumors with specific mutations in the epidermal growth factor receptor (EGFR) tyrosine kinase have been defined as 'oncogene addicted' to indicate their dependence on EGFR and their high susceptibility to the inhibitory effects induced by EGFR tyrosine kinase inhibitors (EGFR-TKIs; eg, gefitinib, erlotinib, afatinib). The most common *EGFR* mutations include a deletion in exon 19 (del E746_A750) and a point substitution in exon 21 (L858R). During the last few years, eight phase III randomized studies comparing an EGFR-TKI versus platinum-based chemotherapy demonstrated that gefitinib, erlotinib, or afatinib are superior to chemotherapy in terms of response rate, progression-free survival, quality of life, and toxicity profile only in patients harboring activating *EGFR* mutations. Moreover, these mutations are also prognostic of a relatively indolent course of disease, regardless of treatment, as compared with classical NSCLC. Although the vast majority of patients harboring *EGFR* mutations respond to EGFR-TKI treatment, no patient achieves a definitive cure and inevitably acquired resistance occurs. The aim of the present handbook is to summarize the role of *EGFR* mutations in NSCLC and to describe the strategies for treating patients.

# Chapter 1

# Introduction

Lung cancer is the most lethal disease in Western countries, with a case mortality rate of 85% [1]. The combination of high incidence and mortality makes lung cancer the leading cause of cancer-related deaths worldwide and it is estimated that it is responsible for more deaths than colorectal, breast, and prostate cancer combined [1]. Non-small cell lung cancer (NSCLC) accounts for 75% of all lung cancers and is divided into different subtypes (adenocarcinoma, squamous cell carcinoma, large cell carcinoma), underlying relevant biological differences (Figure 1.1). Disease stage is the most relevant factor influencing mortality. Approximately 70–80% of patients with NSCLC present with locally advanced or metastatic disease and median survival is approximately 12 months with standard chemotherapy.

The pathogenesis of lung cancer involves the accumulation of several molecular abnormalities over time. Alterations in gene sequence or expression can occur in the cell-signaling and regulatory pathways involved in cell cycle control, apoptosis, proteasome regulation, and angiogenesis. Genetic changes include mutations, gene silencing, gene amplification or deletion, and whole chromosome gains or losses. Lung adenocarcinoma has been extensively investigated and during the last 10 years several molecular events have been discovered leading to a dramatic change in patient treatment [3–7]. Drugs targeting the tyrosine-kinase domain of the epidermal growth factor receptor (EGFR), such as gefitinib, erlotinib, or afatinib, demonstrated superiority versus standard chemotherapy in patients harboring activating *EGFR* mutations [8–13], and crizotinib is

© Springer International Publishing Switzerland 2014
F. Cappuzzo, *Guide to Targeted Therapies: EGFR
mutations in NSCLC*, DOI 10.1007/978-3-319-03059-3_1

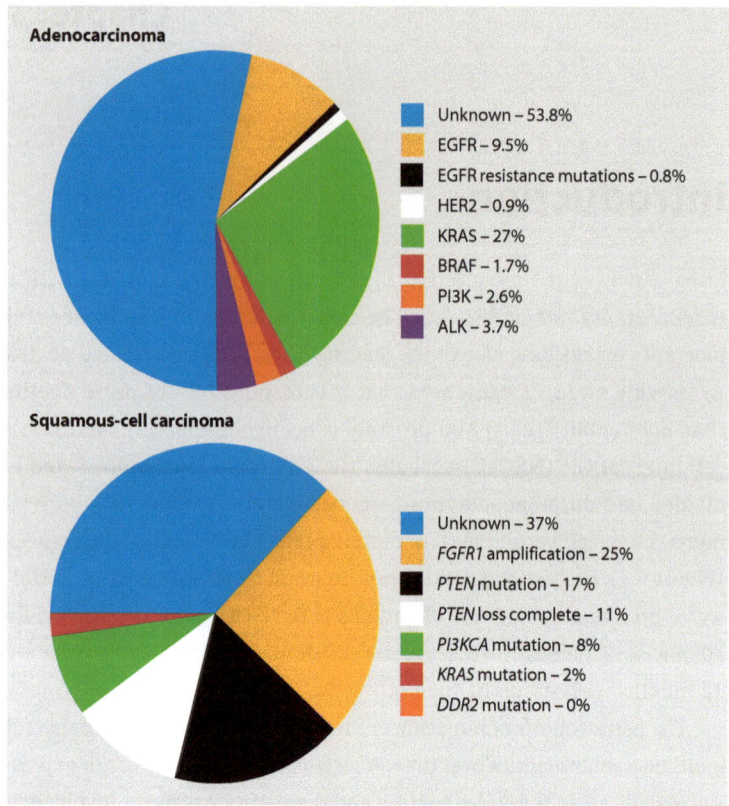

**Figure 1.1 Molecular events in lung cancer.** ALK, anaplastic lymphoma kinase; FGFR, fibroblast growth factor receptor; HER2, human epidermal growth factor receptor 2; PI3K, phosphatidylinositol 3'-kinase; PTEN, phosphatase and tensin homolog. Reproduced with permission from © Barlesi F, Blons H, Beau-Faller M, et al; French Thoracic Intergroup (IFCT). Biomarkers (BM) France: Results of routine EGFR, HER2, KRAS, BRAF, PIK3CA mutations detection and EML4-ALK gene fusion assessment on the first 10,000 non-small cell lung cancer (NSCLC) patients (pts). Slides presented at: 2013 ASCO Annual Meeting; May 31-June 4, 2013; Chicago, IL. Abstract 8000 [2].

now FDA approved for patients with *anaplastic lymphoma kinase (ALK)* translocation [14] (Figure 1.2).

EGFR tyrosine kinase inhibitors (EGFR-TKIs) are the first targeted agents that received approval for metastatic NSCLC. When used in unselected cases, all EGFR-TKIs showed no [15,16] or modest [17] survival improvement over placebo (Figure 1.3). Retrospective review of patients responding to gefitinib or erlotinib revealed discriminating

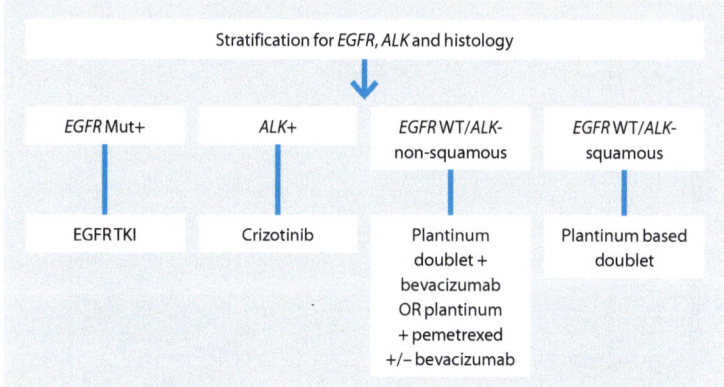

**Figure 1.2 Currently available front-line options for patients with advanced NSCLC.** At the time of this book's publication, front-line therapy for patients with advanced or metastatic NSCLC is based on EGFR and ALK status and on tumor histology. For patients harboring activating *EGFR* mutations, an EGFR-TKI represents the optimal first-line option, as well as crizotinib for patients with ALK translocations. In patients with *EGFR* and *ALK* wild-type mutations, chemotherapy remains the option of choice, with the possibility of using pemetrexed and/or bevacizumab in addition to platinum in non-squamous histology. ALK, anaplastic lymphoma kinase; TKI, tyrosine kinase inhibitor; WT, wild type.

clinical characteristics, including adenocarcinoma histology, never smoking status, female gender, and Asiatic race [19,20]. Nevertheless, all these characteristics were insufficiently sensitive or specific to use in clinical practice to determine which patients might respond to EGFR-TKI therapy. During the last 10 years, several investigators conducted studies to find a suitable biomarker within the tumor to predict which patients were likely to respond to gefitinib or erlotinib and several candidates emerged, including *EGFR* expression [21], *EGFR* gene copy number [22], and *EGFR* mutations [4,5]. It is now clear that *EGFR* mutations represent the most relevant predictor for response to erlotinib, gefitinib, and afatinib with modest and questionable efficacy for such agents in the *EGFR* wild-type population; for example, Mitsudomi et al treated selected patients with gefitinib or cisplatin plus docetaxel, and found that these selected patients with *EGFR* positive mutations had longer progression-free survival on gefitinib than chemotherapy (median progression-free survival was 9.2 months [95% CI 8.0–13.9] in the gefitinib group and 6.3 months [5.8–7.8] in the cisplatin plus docetaxel group [*P*<0.0001]; Figure 1.4) [9]. However, unfortunately, not all patients with *EGFR*

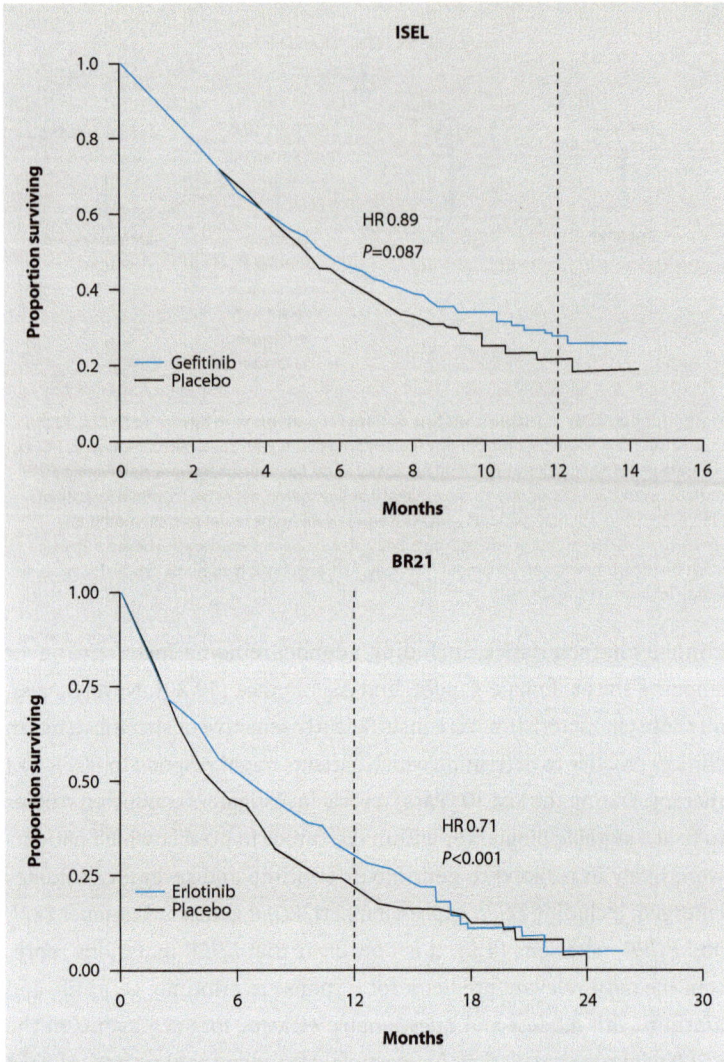

**Figure 1.3 Survival with gefitinib or erlotinib versus placebo in unselected patients with NSCLC.** Two large phase III trials evaluated the efficacy of gefitinib or erlotinib versus placebo in chemotherapy pretreated NSCLC. In EGFR unselected patients, the survival benefit produced by gefitinib or erlotinib was modest and statistically significant only in the erlotinib trial. ISEL, Iressa Survival Evaluation in Lung Cancer study. Reproduced with permission from © Elsevier, 2014; Thatcher et al [15]. Reproduced with permission from © Shepherd et al [18].

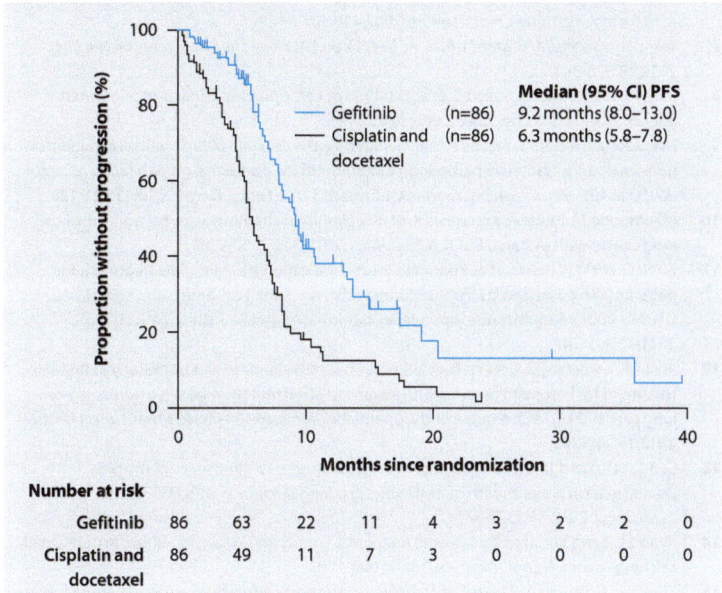

**Figure 1.4 Progression-free survival in untreated patients with NSCLC harboring an activating mutation of the *EGFR* gene.** *P*<0.0001. PFS, progression-free survival. Reproduced with permission from © Elsevier Limited, 2014; Mitsudomi et al [9].

mutations respond to the treatment and inevitably all patients relapse after an initial response to the targeted agent.

The aim of the present review is to summarize the role of *EGFR* mutations and to describe current and future strategies for patients with *EGFR*-dependent NSCLC.

## References

1   DeSantis C, Naishadham D, Jemal A, et al. Cancer statistics for African Americans, 2013. *CA Cancer J Clin*. 2013;63:151-166.
2   Barlesi F, Blons H, Beau-Faller M, et al; French Thoracic Intergroup (IFCT). Biomarkers (BM) France: Results of routine EGFR, HER2, KRAS, BRAF, PI3KCA mutations detection and EML4-ALK gene fusion assessment on the first 10,000 non-small cell lung cancer (NSCLC) patients (pts). Slides presented at: 2013 ASCO Annual Meeting; May 31-June 4, 2013; Chicago, IL. Abstract 8000.
3   Govindan R, Ding L, Griffith M, et al. Genomic landscape of non-small cell lung cancer in smokers and never-smokers. *Cell*. 2012;150:1121-1134.
4   Lynch TJ, Bell DW, Sordella R, et al. Activating mutations in the epidermal growth factor receptor underlying responsiveness of non-small-cell lung cancer to gefitinib. *N Engl J Med*. 2004;350:2129-2139.
5   Paez JG, Jänne PA, Lee JC, et al. EGFR mutations in lung cancer: Correlation with clinical response to gefitinib therapy. *Science*. 2004;304:1497-1500.

6    Soda M, Choi YL, Enomoto M, et al. Identification of the transforming EML4-ALK fusion gene in non-small-cell lung cancer. *Nature*. 2007;448:561-566.

7    Takeuchi K, Soda M, Togashi Y, et al. RET, ROS1 and ALK fusions in lung cancer. *Nat Med*. 2012;18:378-381.

8    Mok TS, Wu YL, Thongprasert S, et al. Gefitinib or carboplatin-paclitaxel in pulmonary adenocarcinoma. *N Engl J Med*. 2009;361:947-957.

9    Mitsudomi T, Morita S, Yatabe Y, et al. Gefitinib versus cisplatin plus docetaxel in patients with non-small cell lung cancer harbouring mutations of the epidermal growth factor receptor (WJTOG3405): An open label, randomised phase 3 trial. *Lancet Oncol*. 2010;11:121-128.

10   Maemondo M, Inoue A, Kobayashi K, et al. Gefitinib or chemotherapy for non–small-cell lung cancer with mutated EGFR. *N Engl J Med*. 2010;362:2380-2388.

11   Zhou C, Wu YL, Chen G, et al. Erlotinib versus chemotherapy as first-line treatment for patients with advanced EGFR mutation-positive non-small cell lung cancer (OPTIMAL, CTONG-0802): A multicentre, open-label, randomised, phase 3 study. *Lancet Oncol*. 2011;12:735-742.

12   Rosell R, Carcereny E, Gervais R, et al. Erlotinib versus standard chemotherapy as first-line treatment for European patients with advanced EGFR mutation-positive non-small-cell lung cancer (EURTAC): A multicentre, open-label, randomised phase 3 trial. *Lancet Oncol*. 2012;13:239-246.

13   Sequist LV, Yang JC, Yamamoto N, et al. Phase III study of afatinib or cisplatin plus pemetrexed in patients with metastatic lung adenocarcinoma with EGFR mutations. *J Clin Oncol*. 2012;31:3327-3334.

14   Kwak EL, Bang YJ, Camidge DR, et al. Anaplastic lymphoma kinase inhibition in non–small-cell lung cancer. *N Engl J Med*. 2010;363:1693-1703.

15   Thatcher N, Chang A, Parikh P, et al. Gefitinib plus best supportive care in previously treated patients with refractory advanced non-small-cell lung cancer: results from a randomised, placebo-controlled, multicentre study (Iressa Survival Evaluation in Lung Cancer). *Lancet*. 2005;366:1527-1537.

16   Miller VA, Hirsh V, Cadranel J, et al. Afatinib versus placebo for patients with advanced, metastatic non-small-cell lung cancer after failure of erlotinib, gefitinib, or both, and one or two lines of chemotherapy (LUX-Lung 1): a phase 2b/3 randomised trial. *Lancet Oncol*. 2012;13:528-538.

17   Shepherd FA, Rodrigues PJ, Ciuleanu T, et al. Erlotinib in previously treated non-small-cell lung cancer. *N Engl J Med*. 2005;353:123-132.

18   Shepherd FA, Pereira J, Ciuleanu T, et al; National Cancer Institute of Canada Clinical Trials Group. A randomized placebo controlled study of erlotinib (OSI-774, Tarceva™) versus placebo in patients with incurable non-small cell lung cancer who have failed standard therapy for advanced or metastatic disease. Slides presented at 2004 ASCO Annual Meeting; June 5-June 7, 2004; New Orleans, LA.

19   Fukuoka M, Yano S, Giaccone G, et al. Multi-institutional randomized phase II trial of gefitinib for previously treated patients with advanced non-small-cell lung cancer. *J Clin Oncol*. 2003;21:2237-2246.

20   Kris MG, Natale RB, Herbst RS, et al. Efficacy of gefitinib, an inhibitor of the epidermal growth factor receptor tyrosine kinase, in symptomatic patients with non-small cell lung cancer: a randomized trial. *JAMA*. 2003;290:2149-2158.

21   Tsao MS, Sakurada A, Cutz JC, et al. Erlotinib in lung cancer molecular and clinical predictors of outcome. *N Engl J Med*. 2005;353:133-144.

22   Cappuzzo F, Hirsch FR, Rossi E, et al. Epidermal growth factor receptor gene and protein and gefitinib sensitivity in non-small-cell lung cancer. *J Natl Cancer Inst*. 2005;97:643-655.

# Chapter 2

# The Human Epidermal growth factor Receptor (HER) family: structure and function

Epidermal growth factor receptor (EGFR) belongs to a family of four different receptors, including EGFR (ErbB-1; human epidermal growth factor receptor 1 [HER1]), HER2 (c-ErbB-2), HER3 (c-ErbB-3), and HER4 (c-ErbB-4). These proteins are coded by distinct genes that are expressed on chromosomes 7, 17, 12, and 2, respectively. Although specific soluble ligands have been identified for the extracellular domains of EGFR, HER3, and HER4, no ligand has been identified for HER2. Several ligands can bind to EGFR, including epidermal growth factor (EGF) and transforming growth factor α (TGFα). After the ligand binds the receptor, the receptor dimerizes, either as a homodimer or as a heterodimer preferentially with HER2, but also with other members of the EGFR family, and undergoes autophosphorylation at specific tyrosine residues within the intracellular domain. These autophosphorylation events in turn activate downstream signaling pathways, including the Ras/Raf/mitogen-activated protein kinase (MAPK) pathway, and the phosphatidylinositol 3'-kinase (PI3K)-Akt pathway. Activation of Ras initiates a multistep phosphorylation cascade that leads to the activation of MAPKs. The MAPKs, ERK1, and ERK2 subsequently regulate gene transcription, and have been linked to cell proliferation, survival, and transformation in laboratory studies [1].

Heterodimerization of EGFR and HER2 is an important mechanism of oncogenic transformation in various tumor types. An NIH3T3 cell line

© Springer International Publishing Switzerland 2014
F. Cappuzzo, *Guide to Targeted Therapies: EGFR mutations in NSCLC*, DOI 10.1007/978-3-319-03059-3_2

devoid of expression of HER family members was used to evaluate the potency of various HER heterodimers for induction of tumor growth by transfecting various combinations of HER proteins [2]. Cells expressing HER2, HER3, or HER4 homodimers were not able to induce tumor growth, whereas cells expressing EGFR had only modest oncogenic properties. HER2/HER3 coexpression was capable of inducing tumor growth, while combinations of HER1/HER3 and HER1/HER4 did not. Conversely, EGFR/HER2 heterodimers were the only HER dimers inducing an aggressive tumorigenic phenotype (Figure 2.1).

EGFR and HER2 are overexpressed in many solid tumors, including lung, head and neck, breast, kidney, colon, ovary, prostate, brain, and bladder cancers [3–5]. Co-overexpression of EGFR and HER2 potentiates the biologic effect of EGFR and it is associated with the highest

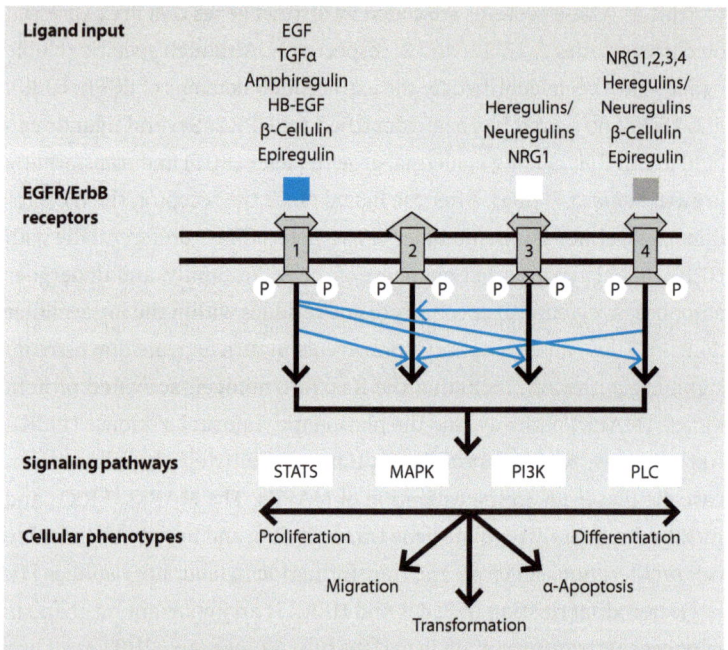

**Figure 2.1 The diversity of the EGFR signaling network.** ErbB, estrogen receptor (tyrosine kinase family) type B; MAPK, mitogen-activated protein kinase; NRG, neuregulin; PI3K, phosphatidylinositol 3'-kinase; PLC, phospholipase C; STATs, signal transducers and activators of transcription; TGFα, transforming growth factor alpha. Reproduced with permission from © Elsevier Limited 2014, Grandis et al [3].

expression of proliferation markers [6]. Because of its enhanced ability to form heterodimers with other HER family members, HER2 represents the preferred dimerization partner for all of the HER receptors [5]. The mechanism by which HER2 amplifies the mitogenic effect of EGFR is likely heterodimerization [6].

## Mechanisms for EGFR deregulation

In non-small cell lung cancer (NSCLC), EGFR is often deregulated. The most frequent events responsible for EGFR deregulation are protein overexpression, gene copy number amplification, or gene mutation (Figure 2.2).

### EGFR overexpression

EGFR protein overexpression is seen in up to 85% of patients with NSCLC, although the prognostic relevance of EGFR expression in this disease remains equivocal [7,8]. EGFR expression assessed by immunohisto-chemistry (IHC) has been the first biological marker to be retrospectively explored in cohorts of patients with NSCLC treated with EGFR tyrosine

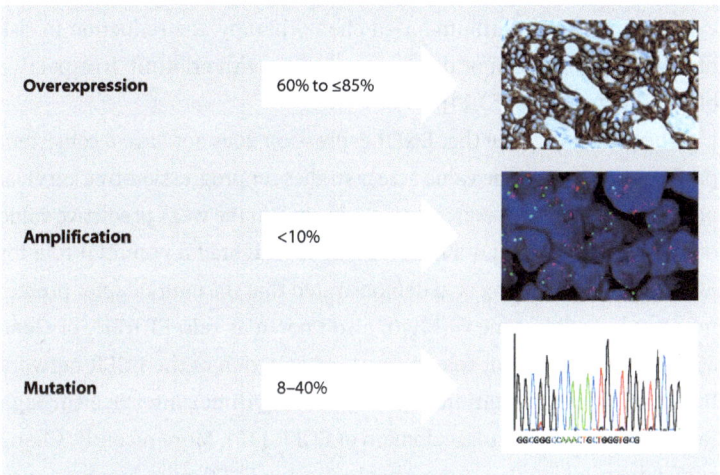

**Figure 2.2 EGFR deregulation in patients with lung cancer.** The most frequent events responsible for EGFR deregulation are protein overexpression (occurring in up to 85% of cases), *EGFR* gene amplification (reported in up to 10% of patients), and *EGFR* mutations (reported in approximately 10% of Caucasian patients and in up to 40% of Asian patients).

kinase inhibitors (EGFR-TKI). Initial retrospective reports showed no association between EGFR levels and tumor response [9,10]. Two large randomized placebo-controlled phase III trials (BR21 and Iressa Survival Evaluation in Lung Cancer study [ISEL]) evaluated the outcome of patients treated with erlotinib or gefitinib, according to EGFR expression. In the BR21 study [11], 325 tumor samples had undergone IHC staining to assess EGFR protein expression. EGFR-IHC positive patients treated with erlotinib had a significant survival improvement when compared with EGFR-IHC positive patients who received placebo (hazard ratio [HR] 0.68, 95% CI 0.49–0.95, $P=0.02$), while no difference was observed among EGFR-IHC negative patients irrespective of treatment delivered (HR 0.93, 95% CI 0.63–1.36, $P=0.70$). Nevertheless, a formal comparison of these HRs indicated that the difference was not significant ($P=0.25$). Conversely, in the ISEL trial [12], EGFR-IHC positive individuals treated with gefitinib had better survival compared with those treated with placebo (HR=0.77, 95% CI 0.56–1.08, $P=0.126$), with a significant interaction test ($P=0.049$). In the Sequential Tarceva in Unresectable NSCLC (SATURN) trial, a large phase III study comparing erlotinib versus placebo as maintenance therapy in patients not progressing after four cycles of first-line platinum-based chemotherapy, the reduction in risk of disease progression or death was similar with erlotinib irrespective of EGFR expression [13,14].

These data indicate that EGFR expression does not have a consistent predictive or prognostic value across studies for progression-free survival or overall survival. Several factors could explain the weak predictive value of EGFR expression and a recent study highlighted a potential role for EGFR regulators. Zhang et al demonstrated that the multiadaptor protein mitogen-inducible gene 6 (Mig6, also known as ralt, ERRFI1, or Gene 33) plays an important role in signal attenuation of the EGFR network by blocking the formation of the activating dimer interface through interaction with the kinase domain of EGFR [15]. More recently, Chang et al demonstrated that tumors not harboring *EGFR* mutations are sensitive to the inhibitory effects of erlotinib in presence of low Mig6/EGFR expression ratio [16], highlighting a potential role for protein expression evaluated by IHC for the identification of *EGFR* wild-type individuals potentially benefiting from an EGFR-TKI treatment.

### *EGFR* gene copy number

Another mechanism responsible for EGFR deregulation is gene amplification. *EGFR* amplification is reported in approximately 10% of cases with an additional 20% of patients displaying high levels of polysomy [17,18] (Figure 2.3). Different studies evaluated the prognostic impact of *EGFR* gene copy number determined by fluorescence in situ hybridization (FISH), and all showed no association with patient survival [18–21]. In our experience while studying a large cohort of patients with surgically resected NSCLC, no difference in survival was observed in patients

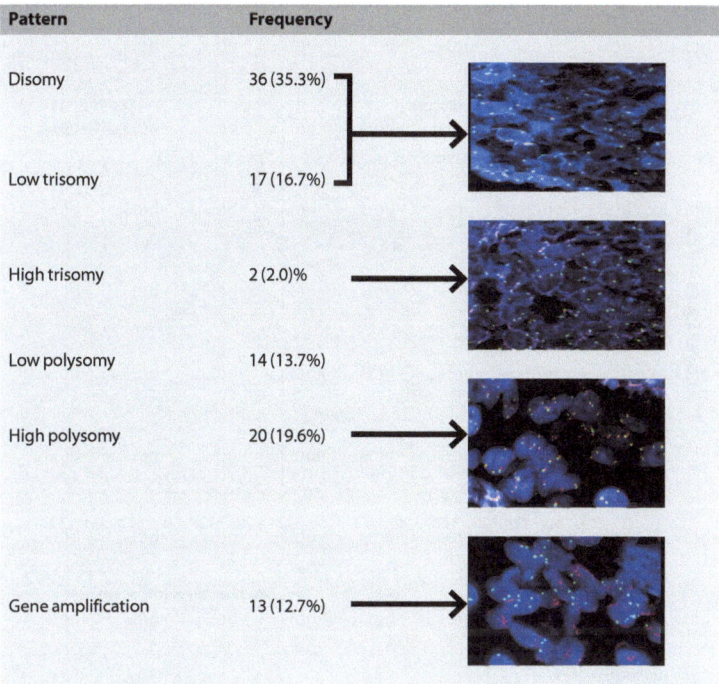

| Pattern | Frequency |
|---|---|
| Disomy | 36 (35.3%) |
| Low trisomy | 17 (16.7%) |
| High trisomy | 2 (2.0)% |
| Low polysomy | 14 (13.7%) |
| High polysomy | 20 (19.6%) |
| Gene amplification | 13 (12.7%) |

**Figure 2.3 *EGFR* gene patterns (fluorescence in situ hybridization).** This figure shows EGFR status according to ascending gene copy number. *EGFR* gene amplification is reported in approximately 10% of cases, with additional 20% of patients with high polysomy. Adapted from Cappuzzo et al [17].

with or without gene amplification, nor when the analysis also included individuals with *EGFR* high polysomy [18], as illustrated in Figure 2.4.

Several studies have investigated the predictive implications of *EGFR* gene copy number evaluated by FISH on sensitivity to EGFR-TKIs. In the first study [17], individuals with *EGFR* high polysomy or gene amplification (defined as *EGFR FISH* positive) had a significantly higher response rate, with a significantly longer time to progression and survival than patients with no *EGFR* gene gain (defined as *EGFR FISH* negative). In the randomized placebo-controlled phase III study of erlotinib versus placebo [11], *EGFR FISH* positive patients treated with erlotinib had a higher response rate and longer survival than *EGFR FISH* positive patients treated with placebo (HR 0.44, 95% CI 0.23–0.82, *P*=0.008), whereas erlotinib offered no advantage in *FISH* negative patients. An update of the same

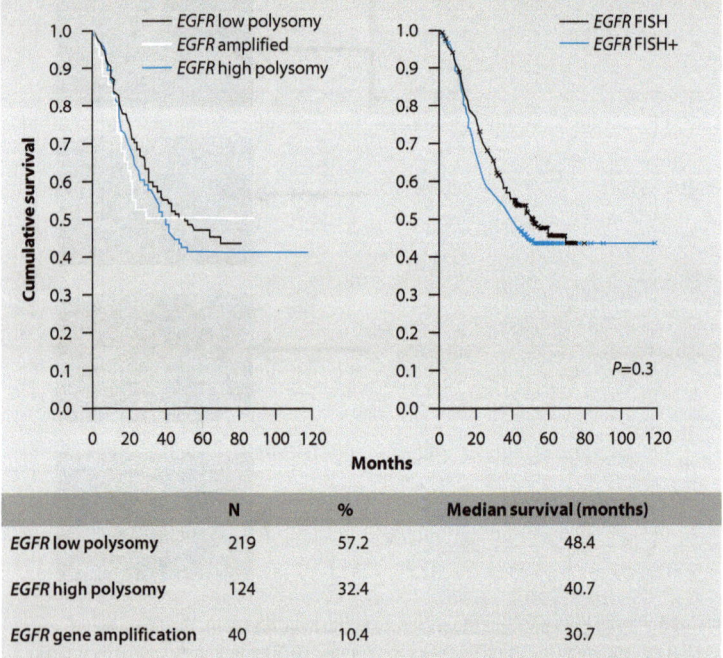

|                          | N   | %    | Median survival (months) |
|--------------------------|-----|------|--------------------------|
| *EGFR* low polysomy      | 219 | 57.2 | 48.4                     |
| *EGFR* high polysomy     | 124 | 32.4 | 40.7                     |
| *EGFR* gene amplification| 40  | 10.4 | 30.7                     |

**Figure 2.4 *EGFR* copy number and survival in patients with NSCLC.** A retrospective analysis of surgically resected NSCLC showed that *EGFR* amplification is not prognostic in resected NSCLC. FISH, fluorescence in situ hybridization. Reproduced with permission from © Cappuzzo et al [18,22].

trial confirmed a significant survival advantage for *EGFR FISH* positive patients treated with erlotinib versus placebo, with a HR of 0.43 [23]. The ISEL trial [12] confirmed the better outcome in terms of response rate and survival for *EGFR FISH* positive patients treated with gefitinib than *EGFR FISH* positive patients treated with placebo, with no survival difference observed between the two arms in *EGFR FISH* patients. The ONCOBELL trial, a prospective phase II study evaluating response rate in *EGFR FISH* positive or never-smoker patients treated with gefitinib confirmed that *EGFR FISH* testing is useful for patient selection [24]. In this study, response rate was 68% in *EGFR FISH* positive and no response was observed in never smokers negative for *EGFR FISH* and mutation.

Nevertheless, two studies mitigated the enthusiasm around FISH testing [25,26]. The Iressa Pan-Asia Study (IPASS) study was a large phase III study that randomly assigned Asian patients with lung adenocarcinoma and who were nonsmokers or former light smokers to front-line therapy with gefitinib or carboplatin plus paclitaxel chemotherapy [27]. In the whole study population gefitinib significantly prolonged progression-free survival versus chemotherapy. Progression-free survival was significantly longer for patients receiving gefitinib whose tumors had both high *EGFR* gene copy number and *EGFR* mutation (HR 0.48, 95% CI 0.34–0.67), but it was significantly shorter when high *EGFR* gene copy number was not accompanied by *EGFR* mutation (HR 3.85, 95% CI 2.09–7.09), indicating that the predictive value of *EGFR* gene copy number was driven by coexisting *EGFR* mutation [25]. The SATURN trial was a large phase III study comparing erlotinib versus placebo in patients with NSCLC not progressing after four cycles of standard first-line platinum-based chemotherapy [13]. The study demonstrated that maintenance erlotinib significantly prolonged progression-free survival and overall survival irrespective of any clinical or biological characteristic, with patients with *EGFR* mutations deriving the highest progression-free survival benefit [13,26]. Erlotinib also produced a significant progression-free survival benefit in patients with *EGFR FISH* positive tumors (HR 0.68, 95% CI 0.51–0.90, $P=0.35$), but no statistically significant benefit in those patients with *EGFR FISH* negative tumors (HR 0.81, 95% CI 0.62–1.07, $P<0.001$) [26]. The interaction between treatment and *EGFR FISH* status was not significant ($P=0.35$). Overall, available data indicate that *EGFR* gene copy number is not an optimal biomarker for guiding selection of patients with NSCLC for EGFR-TKI therapy.

## *EGFR* mutations

The identification of clinical subsets of patients that are more likely to derive a clinical benefit from gefitinib or erlotinib led investigators to further explore EGFR biology. A milestone in driving future strategies for EGFR-TKI development was realized with the discovery of mutations in the EGFR tyrosine kinase domain of patients responding to EGFR-TKIs [28–30], with preclinical data suggesting that *EGFR* mutant lung cancers are EGFR-addicted for tumor growth [29]. These mutations were somatic and more frequently observed in patients with certain clinical features known to be associated with TKI sensitivity, such as female gender, adenocarcinoma histology, Asian ethnicity, and never smoking history. In addition, Pham et al observed that the likelihood of harboring *EGFR* mutations in lung adenocarcinomas decreases as the exposure to tobacco smoke increases [31]. Mutations were less common in people who smoked for more than 15 pack-years or who stopped smoking cigarettes less than 25 years ago. The most common *EGFR* sensitizing mutations, accounting for approximately 85% of all *EGFR* mutations in NSCLC, include deletions in exon 19 and L858 substitutions in exon 21. Such *EGFR* mutations increase sensitivity to TKIs, most likely through induction of critical structural modifications of the adenosine triphosphate (ATP)-binding site in the tyrosine kinase domain [28,29]. Several other *EGFR* gene mutations have been described but their role is not clear, and it is not possible to exclude the possibility that some of them are artifacts [32]. Rare *EGFR* mutations [33] include insertions in exons 19 (1%) and 20 (4%), point mutations in exon 18 (G719: 3%) and in exon 21 (L861: 2%). The most frequent *EGFR* mutations are located within or are related to the ATP-binding site of the kinase, but rare mutations can be localized in other regions of the tyrosine kinase domain (Figure 2.5). For this reason, the correlation between mutation status and response to EGFR-TKI treatment in patients with rare *EGFR* mutations may be different to that observed in patients harboring classical mutations.

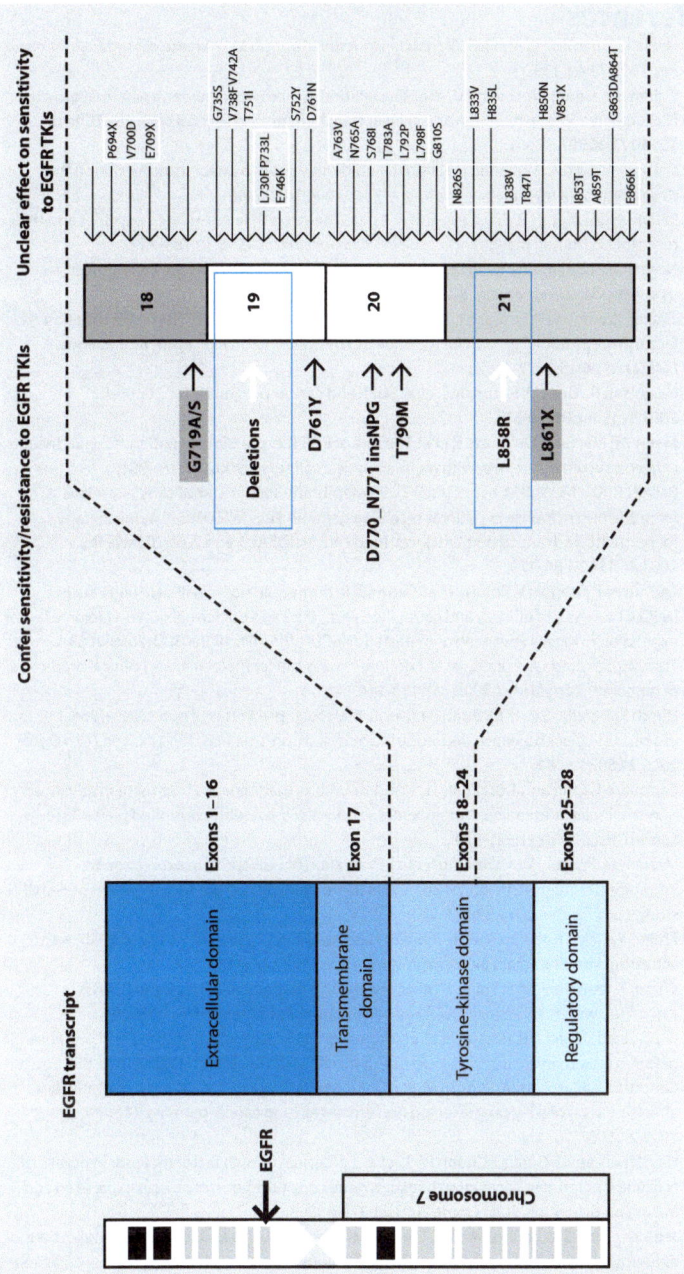

**Figure 2.5 Mutations in the *EGFR* gene.** Mutations in exon 19 or in exon 21 are the most frequent *EGFR* mutations. Additional mutations are reported in other exons. Mutations in exon 20 are generally associated with resistance to gefitinib, erlotinib, or afatinib therapy. TKI, tyrosine kinase inhibitors. Adapted from Riely et al [34].

# References

1   Lewis TS, Shapiro PS, Ahn NG. Signal transduction through MAP kinase cascades. *Adv Cancer Res.* 1998;74:49-139.

2   Cohen BD, Kiener PA, Green JM, et al. The relationship between human epidermal growth-like factor receptor expression and cellular transformation in NIH3T3 cells. *J Biol Chem.* 1996;271:30897-30903.

3   Grandis JR, Sok JC. Signaling through the epidermal growth factor receptor during the development of malignancy. *Pharmacol Ther.* 2004;102:37-46.

4   Salomon DS, Brandt R, Ciardiello F, et al. Epidermal growth factor-related peptides and their receptors in human malignancies. *Crit Rev Oncol Hematol.* 1995;19:183-232.

5   Normanno N, Bianco C, Strizzi L, et al. The ErbB receptors and their ligands in cancer: an overview. *Curr Drug Targets.* 2005;6:243-257.

6   Pinkas-Kramarski R, Soussan L, Waterman H, et al. Diversification of Neu differentiation factor and epidermal growth factor signaling by combinatorial receptor interactions. *EMBO J.* 1996;15:2452-2467.

7   Nicholson RI, Gee JM, Harper ME, et al. EGFR and cancer prognosis. *Eur J Cancer.* 2001;37 (Suppl 4):S9-S15.

8   Meert AP, Martin B, Delmotte P, et al. The role of EGF-R expression on patient survival in lung cancer: a systematic review with meta-analysis. *Eur Respir J.* 2002;20:975-981.

9   Bailey LR, Kris M, Wolf M, et al. Tumor EGFR membrane staining is not clinically relevant for predicting response in patients receiving gefitinib ('Iressa', ZD1839) monotherapy for pretreated advanced non-small-cell lung cancer: IDEAL 1 and 2. *Clin Cancer Res.* 2003;44:1362, LBA-170.

10  Cappuzzo F, Gregorc V, Rossi E, et al. Gefitinib in pretreated non-small-cell lung cancer (NSCLC): analysis of efficacy and correlation with HER2 and epidermal growth factor receptor expression in locally advanced or metastatic NSCLC. *J Clin Oncol.* 2003;21:2658-2663.

11  Tsao MS, Sakurada A, Cutz JC, et al. Erlotinib in lung cancer molecular and clinical predictors of outcome. *N Engl J Med.* 2005;353:133-144.

12  Hirsch Fr, Varella-Garcia M, Bunn Pa Jr, et al. Molecular predictors of outcome with gefitinib in a phase III placebo-controlled study in advanced non-small-cell lung cancer. *J Clin Oncol.* 2006;24:5034-5042.

13  Cappuzzo F, Ciuleanu T, Stelmakh L, et al. Erlotinib as maintenance treatment in advanced non-small-cell lung cancer: a multicentre, randomised, placebo-controlled phase 3 study. *Lancet Oncol.* 2010;11:521-529.

14  Mazières J, Brugger W, Cappuzzo F, et al. Evaluation of EGFR protein expression by immunohistochemistry using H-score and the magnification rule: re-analysis of the SATURN study. *Lung Cancer.* 2013;82:231-237.

15  Zhang X, Pickin KA, Bose R, et al. Inhibition of the EGF receptor by binding of MIG6 to an activating kinase domain interface. *Nature.* 2007;450:741-744.

16  Chang X, Izumchenko E, Solis LM, et al. The relative expression of Mig6 and EGFR is associated with resistance to EGFR kinase inhibitors. *PLoS One.* 2013;8:e68966.

17  Cappuzzo F, Hirsch FR, Rossi E, et al. Epidermal growth factor receptor gene and protein and gefitinib sensitivity in non-small-cell lung cancer. *J Natl Cancer Inst.* 2005;97:643-655.

18  Cappuzzo F, Marchetti A, Skokan M, et al. Increased MET gene copy number negatively affects survival of surgically resected non-small-cell lung cancer patients. *J Clin Oncol.* 2009;27:1667-1674.

19  Hirsch FR, Varella-Garcia M, Bunn PA Jr, et al. Epidermal growth factor receptor in non-small-cell lung carcinomas: correlation between gene copy number and protein expression and impact on prognosis. *J Clin Oncol.* 2003;21:3798-3807.

20  Jeon YK, Sung SW, Chung JH, et al. Clinicopathologic features and prognostic implications of epidermal growth factor receptor (EGFR) gene copy number and protein expression in non-small cell lung cancer. *Lung Cancer.* 2006;54:387-398.

21    Suzuki S, Dobashi Y, Sakurai H, et al. Protein overexpression and gene amplification of epidermal growth factor receptor in non small cell lung carcinomas. An immunohistochemical and fluorescence in situ hybridization study. *Cancer*. 2005;103:1265-1273.

22    Cappuzzo F, Skokan M, Gajapathy S, et al. Effect of increased MET gene copy number on survival of surgically resected non-small cell lung cancer (NSCLC) patients. Data presented at the 2008 ASCO Annual Meeting; May 30-June 1, 2008. Abstract 11047.

23    Shepherd F, Ding K, Sakurada A, et al. Updated molecular analyses of exons 19 and 21 of the epidermal growth factor receptor (EGFR) gene and codons 12 and 13 of the KRAS gene in non-small cell lung cancer (NSCLC) patients treated with erlotinib in National Cancer Institute of Cancer. *J Clin Oncol*. 2007;25:7571a.

24    Cappuzzo F, Ligorio C, Jänne PA, et al. Prospective study of gefitinib in epidermal growth factor receptor fluorescence in situ hybridization-positive/phospho-Akt-positive or never smoker patients with advanced non-small-cell lung cancer: the ONCOBELL trial. *J Clin Oncol*. 2007;25:2248-2255.

25    Fukuoka M, Wu YL, Thongprasert S, et al. Biomarker analyses and final overall survival results from a phase III, randomized, open-label, first-line study of gefitinib versus carboplatin/paclitaxel in clinically selected patients with advanced non-small-cell lung cancer in Asia (IPASS). *J Clin Oncol*. 2011;29:2866-2874.

26    Brugger W, Triller N, Blasinska-Morawiec M, et al. Prospective molecular marker analyses of EGFR and KRAS from a randomized, placebo-controlled study of erlotinib maintenance therapy in advanced non-small-cell lung cancer. *J Clin Oncol*. 2011;29:4113-4120.

27    Mok TS, Wu YL, Thongprasert S, et al. Gefitinib or carboplatin-paclitaxel in pulmonary adenocarcinoma. *N Engl J Med*. 2009;361:947-957.

28    Lynch TJ, Bell DW, Sordella R et al. Activating mutations in the epidermal growth factor receptor underlying responsiveness of non-small-cell lung cancer to gefitinib. *N Engl J Med*. 2004;350:2129-2139.

29    Paez JG, Jänne PA, Lee JC, et al. EGFR mutations in lung cancer: Correlation with clinical response to gefitinib therapy. *Science*. 2004;304:1497-1500.

30    Pao W, Miller V, Zakowski M, et al. EGF receptor gene mutations are common in lung cancers from "never smokers" and are associated with sensitivity of tumors to gefitinib and erlotinib. *PNAS USA*. 2004;101:13306-13311.

31    Pham D, Kris MG, Riely GJ, et al. Use of cigarette-smoking history to estimate the likelihood of mutations in epidermal growth factor receptor gene exons 19 and 21 in lung adenocarcinomas. *J Clin Oncol*. 2006;24:1700-1704.

32    Marchetti A, Felicioni L, Buttitta F, et al. Assessing EGFR mutations. *N Engl J Med*. 2006;354:526-528.

33    Yasuda H, Kobayashi S, Costa DB, et al; EGFR exon 20 insertion mutations in non-small-cell lung cancer: preclinical data and clinical implications. *Lancet Oncol*. 2012;13:e23-e31.

34    Riely GJ, Pao W, Pham D, et al. Clinical course of patients with non-small cell lung cancer and epidermal growth factor receptor exon 19 and exon 21 mutations treated with gefitinib or erlotinib. *Clin Cancer Res*. 2006;12:839-844.

# Chapter 3

# Methods for *EGFR* mutation testing

*Epidermal growth factor receptor (EGFR)* mutations are generally detected in DNA from samples of tumor tissue obtained during biopsy or surgcial resection, usually in the form of formalin-fixed paraffin-embedded (FFPE) diagnostic blocks, using gene sequencing. While this method has been regarded as the gold standard, it has several disadvantages, mainly a low sensitivity, with the consequent risk of missing *EGFR* mutation positive patients [1]. During recent years, several alternative methods for mutation testing have been developed, many with improved sensitivity and turnaround times. Table 3.1 illustrates the main methods for *EGFR* mutation testing.

Searching for alternative methods to direct sequencing, Sueoka et al showed that mutation testing results obtained by denaturing high-performance liquid chromatography (dHPLC) analysis of frozen tissue samples were consistent with those obtained by direct sequencing, with a significant reduction in time analysis [2]. Takano et al showed that high-resolution melting analysis (HRMA) has higher sensitivity and specificity when compared to sequencing [3]. Borras et al reported identical *EGFR* mutation frequency rates to direct sequencing by using HRMA [4]. Querings et al evaluated an alternative next-generation sequencing methodology, the massively parallel sequencing [5]. In this study, the method yielded a 100% success rate to detect low-frequency *EGFR* mutations compared with 67% for direct sequencing, and with 89% for pyrosequencing, a non-electrophoretic sequencing technology employing luminometric detection [5].

© Springer International Publishing Switzerland 2014
F. Cappuzzo, *Guide to Targeted Therapies: EGFR
mutations in NSCLC*, DOI 10.1007/978-3-319-03059-3_3

| Method | Screening technologies | Targeted technologies | Sensitivity (% of mutant DNA) | Comments |
|---|---|---|---|---|
| PCR-sequencing | X | | 20% | Requires at least 50% of neoplastic cell in the sample |
| Pyrosequencing | X | | 5–10% | |
| PCR/dHPLC/HRMA (Melt analysis) | X | | 5% | Only screening for mutation |
| Fragment analysis Genscan – PCR/SSCP | X | | 5% | Only screening for mutation |
| TaQMAn–PCR | | X | 5–10% | |
| SNAPSHOT | | X | 5–10% | |
| Scorpion ARMS | | X | 1% | |
| PNA/LNA clamp | | X | 0.1–1% | |
| ME PCR/sequencing | | X | 0.1–1% | |

**Table 3.1 Methods for EGFR mutation detection.** The table shows the main methods for detecting EGFR mutations, and what type of technology they are (ie, sequencing or targeted technology). Sequencing is the most common method and kits based on the ARMS method are the most widely available commercial kits. More sensitive tests can more likely identify rare mutations. ARMS, Amplified Refractory Mutation System; dHPLC, denaturing high-performance liquid chromatography; HRMA, high-resolution melting analysis; LNA, locked nucleic acid; ME PCR, multithreaded e-polymerase chain reaction; PCR, polymerase chain reaction; SSCP, single-stranded conformational polymorphism.

Additional studies have assessed targeted methods for detection of common EGFR mutations [6–14]. The majority of these studies investigated the use of polymerase chain reaction (PCR)-based methods to specifically detect exon 19 deletions, the exon 21 L858R point mutation, and, in some cases, other less common but known EGFR mutations [6–10]. These studies varied in the use of frozen and/or FFPE tissue samples. These tests were able to detect all the mutations previously detected on the same samples with direct sequencing, but most importantly, targeted methods detected mutations in samples that had shown a negative result with direct sequencing. For example, Ellison et al showed that the Amplification Refractory Mutation System (ARMS), a method that discriminates between mutated and wild-type DNA by selectively amplifying mutation-containing target sequences, was more sensitive than direct sequencing in detecting classical EGFR mutations [7] even if direct sequencing identified additional mutations not detectable by the specific ARMS reactions. In addition, fragment length analysis is another commonly used method showing more sensitivity than direct sequencing in detecting exon 19 deletions [8].

Testing *EGFR* mutations in clinical practice is sometimes difficult for several reasons, including amount and quality of tumor sample, time needed for obtaining results, and available facilities. Certainly, there is a real need for a rapid, sensitive, and low-cost assay for *EGFR* screening. The majority of groups are now using either direct sequencing or the Scorpion ARMS assay for mutation screening and depending on the assay used for *EGFR* mutation screening, the turnaround time can vary with a realistic time of 5–7 working days. Direct sequencing is thought to be less sensitive and more time-consuming than the Scorpion ARMS assay. The Scorpion ARMS assay requires batching of samples, which may cause delays in the turnaround time of the assay. Newer tests, such as *EGFR* mutation-specific antibodies, are promising and are currently under investigation. They might offer the advantage of sparing tissue, which is of extreme importance, given the emergence of other predictive biomarkers. Immunohistochemical (IHC) analysis is also quick, cost-effective, and is routinely carried out in pathology laboratories. Several studies have evaluated the utility of IHC for detecting *EGFR* mutations [15–20]. These studies utilized two mutant-specific rabbit monoclonal antibodies directed against the exon 19 A746_A750 deletion and L858R, and most reported high sensitivity and specificity for mutant-specific IHC versus direct sequencing or other methods.

## Sources for *EGFR* mutation testing

A relevant clinical problem for assessment of *EGFR* mutations consists of obtaining suitable DNA for analysis. The quality of the samples, the quality of the extracted DNA, and the quantity of DNA available using current methods may limit the routine use of genotypic assessment. At the time of this book's publication, the best source for *EGFR* mutation testing is a tumor specimen obtained during curative surgery or diagnostic biopsy. Although surgery offers the best chance of high-quality and high-volume tumor tissue samples, only 20–25% of patients with lung cancer are suitable for curative surgery and EGFR-TKI therapy is only licensed for use in advanced disease. Consequently, in the vast majority of cases, diagnosis is based on the analysis of a small biopsy or on cytological specimens.

Several studies have assessed the feasibility of *EGFR* mutation testing on cytological specimens. Commonly tested cytology samples included specimens collected during diagnosis, including fine-needle aspirate (FNA) samples or liquid-based samples obtained from patients experiencing common complications of lung cancer, such as pleural effusion. Use of sensitive mutation testing methods is warranted when cytology samples with low tumor content are used. Some studies reported that mutant-enriched PCR and the sensitive ARMS technique were able to detect those *EGFR* mutations in pleural effusion samples not identified via direct sequencing [21,22]. The ARMS method was also more sensitive than direct sequencing in studies utilizing transbronchial FNA [23]. Additional techniques used in clinical practice for diagnosis of non-small cell lung cancer (NSCLC) include endobronchial ultrasound-guided (EBUS)-FNA, trans-esophageal ultrasound-guided (EUS)-FNA and CT-guided FNA. Cytology samples obtained via these techniques were successfully assessed for *EGFR* mutations using direct sequencing [24,25], real-time PCR [26,27], COLD-PCR [28], PNA-locked nucleic acid (LNA) PCR clamp [29], or loop-hybrid mobility shift assay [30].

Although these new techniques are improving our ability to detect *EGFR* mutations, in many cases, after completing all the standard diagnostic procedures, there is no material available for biomarker analysis. In such cases a new tumor biopsy should be performed. Several groups are investigating the possibility of performing biomarker analyses, including *EGFR* mutation testing, in circulating tumor cells (CTCs) or in circulating DNA. The ability to accurately detect somatic cancer DNA alterations from CTCs or from cell free circulating plasma tumor DNA (ptDNA) using next generation genomic technologies has many potential applications for clinical oncology. This approach allows us not only to define the mutational status before starting a targeted therapy but also to define the molecular changes occurring in cancer under therapeutic pressure, facilitating the identification of new potentially targetable events. Until recently, it has not been possible to obtain 'pure' CTCs, but only a CTC-enriched fraction [31]. However, a new method developed by Maheswaran et al allows the isolation of CTCs at high purity from almost all samples tested [32]. This method provided sufficient DNA for *EGFR* mutation analysis in 11 out of 12 patients included in the study. Although some groups have seen a 92% detection rate in CTCs, these cells are difficult to detect in NSCLC and further validation of these techniques are necessary before implementation into routine diagnostics.

# References

1   Eberhard DA, Giaccone G, Johnson BE, et al. Biomarkers of response to epidermal growth factor receptor inhibitors in non-small-cell lung cancer working group: standardization for use in the clinical trial setting. *J Clin Oncol*. 2008;26:983-994.

2   Sueoka N, Sato A, Eguchi H, et al. Mutation profile of EGFR gene detected by denaturing high-performance liquid chromatography in Japanese lung cancer patients. *J Cancer Res Clin Oncol*. 2007;133:93-102.

3   Takano T, Ohe Y, Tsuta K, et al. Epidermal growth factor receptor mutation detection using high-resolution melting analysis predicts outcomes in patients with advanced non-small cell lung cancer treated with gefitinib. *Clin Cancer Res*. 2007;13:5385-5390.

4   Borràs E, Jurado I, Hernan I, et al. Clinical pharmacogenomic testing of KRAS, BRAF and EGFR mutations by high resolution melting analysis and ultra-deep pyrosequencing. *BMC Cancer*. 2011;11:406.

5   Querings S, Altmüller J, Ansén S, et al. Benchmarking of mutation diagnostics in clinical lung cancer specimens. *PLoS One*. 2011;6:e19601.

6   Endo K, Konishi A, Sasaki H, et al. Epidermal growth factor receptor gene mutation in non-small cell lung cancer using highly sensitive and fast TaqMan PCR assay. *Lung Cancer*. 2005;50:375-384.

7   Ellison G, Donald E, McWalter G, et al. A comparison of ARMS and DNA sequencing for mutation analysis in clinical biopsy samples. *J Exp Clin Cancer Res*. 2010;29:132.

8   Pan Q, Pao W, Ladanyi M. Rapid polymerase chain reaction-based detection of epidermal growth factor receptor gene mutations in lung adenocarcinomas. *J Mol Diagn*. 2005;7:396-403.

9   Dufort S, Richard MJ, Lantuejoul S, et al. Pyrosequencing, a method approved to detect the two major EGFR mutations for anti EGFR therapy in NSCLC. *J Exp Clin Cancer Res*. 2011;30:57.

10  Yang Q, Qiu T, Wu W, et al. Simple and sensitive method for detecting point mutations of epidermal growth factor receptor using cationic conjugated polymers. *ACS Appl Mater Interfaces*. 2011;3:4539-4545.

11  Miyamae Y, Shimizu K, Mitani Y, et al. Mutation detection of epidermal growth factor receptor and KRAS genes using the Smart Amplification Process version 2 from formalin-fixed, paraffin-embedded lung cancer tissue. *J Mol Diagn*. 2010;12:257-264.

12  Hoshi K, Takakura H, Mitani Y, et al. Rapid detection of epidermal growth factor receptor mutations in lung cancer by the SMart-Amplification Process. *Clin Cancer Res*. 2007;13:4974-4983.

13  Han HS, Lim SN, An JY, et al. Detection of EGFR mutation status in lung adenocarcinoma specimens with different proportions of tumor cells using two methods of differential sensitivity. *J Thorac Oncol*. 2012;7:355-364.

14  Araki T, Shimizu K, Nakamura T, et al. Clinical screening assay for EGFR exon 19 mutations using PNA-clamp smart amplification process version 2 in lung adenocarcinoma. *Oncol Rep*. 2011;26:1213-1219.

15  Kozu Y, Tsuta K, Kohno T, et al. The usefulness of mutation-specific antibodies in detecting epidermal growth factor receptor mutations and in predicting response to tyrosine kinase inhibitor therapy in lung adenocarcinoma. *Lung Cancer*. 2011;73:45-50.

**16**   Brevet M, Arcila M, Ladanyi M, et al. Assessment of EGFR mutation status in lung adenocarcinoma by immunohistochemistry using antibodies specific to the two major forms of mutant EGFR. *J Mol Diagn.* 2010;12:169-176.

**17**   Ilie MI, Hofman V, Bonnetaud C, et al. Usefulness of tissue microarrays for assessment of protein expression, gene copy number and mutational status of EGFR in lung adenocarcinoma. *Virchows Arch.* 2010;457:483-495.

**18**   Kato Y, Peled N, Wynes MW, et al. Novel epidermal growth factor receptor mutation-specific antibodies for non-small cell lung cancer: immunohistochemistry as a possible screening method for epidermal growth factor receptor mutations. *J Thorac Oncol.* 2010;5:1551-1558.

**19**   Nakamura H, Mochizuki A, Shinmyo T, et al. Immunohistochemical detection of mutated epidermal growth factor receptors in pulmonary adenocarcinoma. *Anticancer Res.* 2010;30:5233-5237.

**20**   Simonetti S, Molina MA, Queralt C, et al. Detection of EGFR mutations with mutation-specific antibodies in stage IV non-small-cell lung cancer. *J Transl Med.* 2010;8:135.

**21**   Soh J, Toyooka S, Aoe K, et al. Usefulness of EGFR mutation screening in pleural fluid to predict the clinical outcome of gefitinib treated patients with lung cancer. *Int J Cancer.* 2006;119:2353-2358.

**22**   Kimura H, Fujiwara Y, Sone T, et al. High sensitivity detection of epidermal growth factor receptor mutations in the pleural effusion of non-small cell lung cancer patients. *Cancer Sci.* 2006;97:642-648.

**23**   Horiike A, Kimura H, Nishio K, et al. Detection of epidermal growth factor receptor mutation in transbronchial needle aspirates of non-small cell lung cancer. *Chest.* 2007;131:1628-1634.

**24**   Schuurbiers OCJ, Looijen-Salamon MG, Ligtenberg MJL, et al. A brief retrospective report on the feasibility of epidermal growth factor receptor and KRAS mutation analysis in transesophageal ultrasound- and endobronchial ultrasound-guided fine needle cytological aspirates. *J Thorac Oncol.* 2010;5:1664-1667.

**25**   Zhuang Y-P, Wang H-Y, Shi M-Q, et al. Use of CT-guided fine needle aspiration biopsy in epidermal growth factor receptor mutation analysis in patients with advanced lung cancer. *Acta Radiol.* 2011;52:1083-1087.

**26**   van Eijk R, Licht J, Schrumpf M, et al. Rapid KRAS, EGFR, BRAF and PIK3CA mutation analysis of fine needle aspirates from non-small-cell lung cancer using allele-specific qPCR. *PLoS One.* 2011;6:e17791.

**27**   Navani N, Brown JM, Nankivell M, et al. Suitability of EBUS-TBNA specimens for subtyping and genotyping of NSCLC: a multi-centre study of 774 patients. *Am J Respir Crit Care Med.* 2012;185:1316-1322.

**28**   Santis G, Angell R, Nickless G, et al. Screening for EGFR and KRAS mutations in endobronchial ultrasound derived transbronchial needle aspirates in non-small cell lung cancer using COLD-PCR. *PLoS One.* 2011;6:e25191.

**29**   Nakajima T, Yasufuku K, Nakagawara A, et al. Multigene mutation analysis of metastatic lymph nodes in non-small cell lung cancer diagnosed by endobronchial ultrasound-guided transbronchial needle aspiration. *Chest.* 2011;140:1319-1324.

**30**   Nakajima T, Yasufuku K, Suzuki M, et al. Assessment of epidermal growth factor receptor mutation by endobronchial ultrasound-guided transbronchial needle aspiration. *Chest.* 2007;132:597-602.

**31**   Smirnov DA, Zweitzig DR, Foulk BW, et al. Global gene expression profiling of circulating tumor cells. *Cancer Res.* 2005;65:4993-4997.

**32**   Maheswaran S, Sequist LV, Nagrath S, et al. Detection of mutations in EGFR in circulating lung-cancer cells. *N Engl J Med.* 2008;359:366-377.

# Chapter 4

# Predictive and prognostic implications of *EGFR* mutations

## Prognostic significance of *EGFR* mutations

Several studies have suggested that *epidermal growth factor receptor (EGFR)* mutations are themselves associated with improved prognosis independent of treatment. In the placebo arm of BR21, a phase III study comparing erlotinib versus placebo in second- or third-line therapy in metastatic non-small cell lung cancer (NSCLC), the median survival time was 9.1 months among patients with activating *EGFR* mutations and 3.5 months in those with wild-type *EGFR* [1]. Combined data from patients treated in the TRIBUTE (Tarceva responses in conjunction with pacli-taxel and carboplatin) study [2], a phase III trial comparing carbopla-tin–paclitaxel with or without erlotinib in the front-line setting, revealed significant differences between *EGFR* mutated and *EGFR* wild-type in time to progression (TTP; 8 months versus 5 months; $P<0.001$) and overall survival (not reached versus 10 months; $P<0.001$). In the INTACT 1 and 2 trials, two large phase III studies comparing platinum-based chemo-therapy with or without gefitinib as first-line therapy, patients harboring *EGFR* mutations had longer survival irrespective of treatment received [3,4]. Similarly, in the INTEREST trial (Iressa NSCLC Trial Evaluating REsponse and Survival versus Taxotere)[5], overall survival was signifi-cantly longer among patients with *EGFR* mutations treated with either gefitinib (median 14.2 months) or docetaxel (16.6 months) than in those with wild-type *EGFR* (6.4 months versus 6.0 months, respectively).

© Springer International Publishing Switzerland 2014
F. Cappuzzo, *Guide to Targeted Therapies: EGFR mutations in NSCLC*, DOI 10.1007/978-3-319-03059-3_4

In order to investigate whether the presence of *EGFR* mutations represents a predictive marker for survival benefit from gefitinib or a prognostic
marker in patients with advanced adenocarcinoma, Japanese investigators analyzed the outcome of patients who began first-line chemotherapy
before and after gefitinib approval in Japan [6]. The authors reported a
significantly longer survival among *EGFR* mutant patients treated after
gefitinib approval, when compared with survival of patients harboring
*EGFR* mutations treated before gefitinib approval, whereas no difference
was observed in patients without *EGFR* mutations. Importantly, among
patients treated before gefitinib registration, those with *EGFR* mutations
lived significantly longer than those without *EGFR* mutations. These data
clearly indicate that *EGFR* mutations significantly predict both a survival
benefit from gefitinib therapy and a favorable prognosis in patients with
advanced lung adenocarcinoma.

Recent studies have suggested that presence of the T790M *EGFR*
mutation in tumor specimens collected before or after exposure to
EGFR-tyrosine kinase inhibitors (TKIs) confers better prognosis [7,8].
At least 50% of cases of acquired resistance are attributable to T790M,
a secondary mutation in the exon 20 of EGFR [9–11]. T790M is thought
to negate the effect of TKIs, and it is sometimes detected in patients
who have not yet received TKI therapy [12–17]. Oxnard et al analyzed
93 patients with NSCLC *EGFR* mutations for presence of the secondary
T790M mutation in tumor specimens collected at the time of EGFR-TKI
failure. Interestingly, patients with T790M had a significantly longer survival than patients without T790M, indicating that the presence of T790M
defines a clinical subset with a relatively favorable prognosis and more
indolent progression [7]. Rosell et al analyzed the outcome of patients with
*EGFR* mutations enrolled onto the EURTAC study, a large phase III trial
comparing erlotinib versus platinum-based chemotherapy in untreated
patients with metastatic NSCLC [8]. In this study, patients harboring the
T790M had longer survival irrespective of the treatment, reinforcing the
hypothesis that this mutation represents a favorable prognostic factor.

Conversely, in early stage disease the prognostic role of *EGFR* mutations has not been confirmed. Three different Asiatic studies showed that
*EGFR* mutations do not independently predict survival among patients who

undergo surgical resection of early NSCLC [18–20]. In the study conducted by Kosaka et al, although one univariate analysis of 397 patients found that patients with *EGFR* mutations survived longer than those without mutations, this association disappeared on multivariate analysis [20].

## *EGFR* mutations and sensitivity to chemotherapy

The predictive value of *EGFR* mutations in patients treated with chemotherapy alone remains unclear. According to a retrospective analysis conducted in East Asian patients treated with chemotherapy, *EGFR* mutation was not associated with improved survival as compared with wild-type *EGFR*, despite a non-statistically significant trend toward a higher response rate [21]. In 2007, we analyzed a cohort of 190 patients with NSCLC with the aim of exploring whether *EGFR* expression, gene copy number, or mutation was predictive for sensitivity to first-line chemotherapy in metastatic disease. This retrospective study showed no association between EGFR deregulation and response to chemotherapy, irrespective of the method used for EGFR assessment [22]. In the IPASS study, a significantly higher response rate to chemotherapy was observed in patients harboring *EGFR* mutations [12]. In the INTEREST (Iressa NSCLC Trial Evaluating REsponse and Survival versus Taxotere) study, an impressive 21% response rate was observed in patients with *EGFR* mutations treated with docetaxel as second-line therapy [5]. Among the predominantly white population included in the adjuvant JBR10 trial, the presence of exon 19 deletions or L858R mutations was associated with a non-significant trend towards a survival benefit following adjuvant chemotherapy with vinorelbine and cisplatin [23]. Therefore, based on available data, it is possible that presence of *EGFR* mutations confers higher sensitivity to standard chemotherapy (Table 4.1).

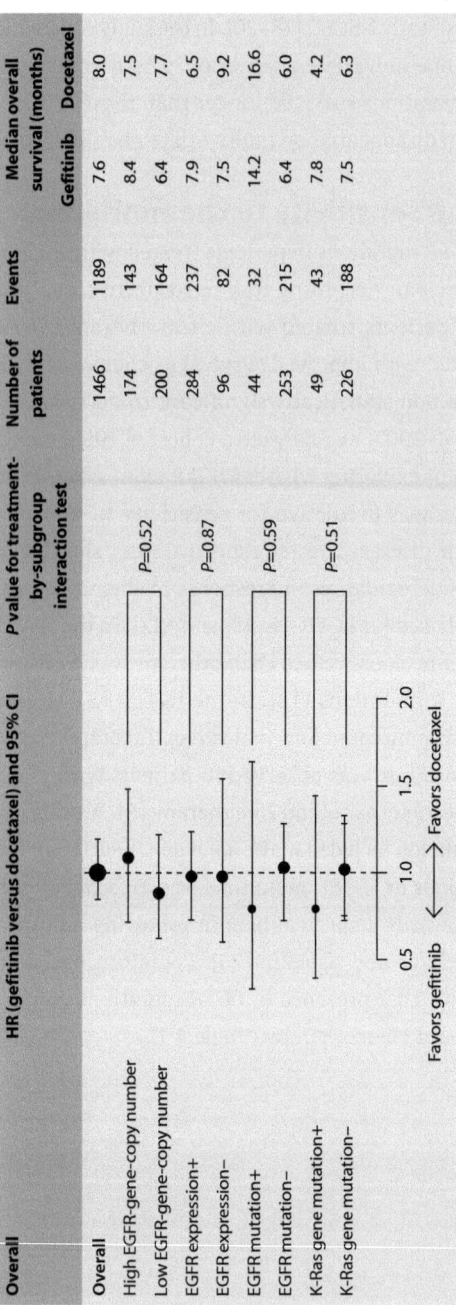

| Overall | HR (gefitinib versus docetaxel) and 95% CI | P value for treatment-by-subgroup interaction test | Number of patients | Events | Median overall survival (months) Gefitinib | Docetaxel |
| --- | --- | --- | --- | --- | --- | --- |
| Overall | | | 1466 | 1189 | 7.6 | 8.0 |
| High EGFR-gene-copy number | | P=0.52 | 174 | 143 | 8.4 | 7.5 |
| Low EGFR-gene-copy number | | | 200 | 164 | 6.4 | 7.7 |
| EGFR expression+ | | P=0.87 | 284 | 237 | 7.9 | 6.5 |
| EGFR expression− | | | 96 | 82 | 7.5 | 9.2 |
| EGFR mutation+ | | P=0.59 | 44 | 32 | 14.2 | 16.6 |
| EGFR mutation− | | | 253 | 215 | 6.4 | 6.0 |
| K-Ras gene mutation+ | | P=0.51 | 49 | 43 | 7.8 | 4.2 |
| K-Ras gene mutation− | | | 226 | 188 | 7.5 | 6.3 |

**Table 4.1 Forest plot of overall survival by biomarkers in the intention-to-treat population.** The INTEREST trial (Iressa NSCLC Trial Evaluating REsponse and Survival versus Taxotere) suggested that chemotherapy is more effective in mutated patients when compared to EGFR wild-type individuals. Reproduced with permission from © Elsevier 2014, Kim et al [24].

# References

1   Shepherd FA, Tsao M. Unraveling the mystery of prognostic and predictive factors in epidermal growth factor receptor therapy. *J Clin Oncol.* 2006;24:1219-1220.

2   Herbst RS, Prager D, Hermann R, et al. TRIBUTE: a phase III trial of erlotinib hydrochloride (OSI-774) combined with carboplatin and paclitaxel chemotherapy in advanced non-small-cell lung cancer. *J Clin Oncol.* 2005;23:5892-5899.

3   Giaccone G, Herbst RS, Manegold C, et al. Gefitinib in combination with gemcitabine and cisplatin in advanced non-small-cell lung cancer: a phase III trial--INTACT 1. *J Clin Oncol.* 2004;22:777-784.

4   Herbst RS, Giaccone G, Schiller JH, et al. Gefitinib in combination with paclitaxel and carboplatin in advanced non-small-cell lung cancer: a phase III trial--INTACT 2. *J Clin Oncol.* 2004;22:785-794.

5   Douillard JY, Shepherd FA, Hirsh V, et al. Molecular predictors of outcome with gefitinib and docetaxel in previously treated non-small-cell lung cancer: data from the randomized phase III INTEREST trial. *J Clin Oncol.* 2010;28:744-752.

6   Takano T, Fukui T, Ohe Y, et al. EGFR mutations predict survival benefit from gefitinib in patients with advanced lung adenocarcinoma: a historical comparison of patients treated before and after gefitinib approval in Japan. *J Clin Oncol.* 2008;26:5589-5595.

7   Oxnard GR, Arcila ME, Sima CS, et al. Acquired resistance to EGFR tyrosine kinase inhibitors in EGFR-mutant lung cancer: distinct natural history of patients with tumors harboring the T790M mutation. *Clin Cancer Res.* 2011;17:1616-1622.

8   Rosell R, Molina-Vila MA, Taron M, et al. EGFR compound mutants and survival on erlotinib in non-small cell lung cancer (NSCLC) patients (p) in the EURTAC study. *J Clin Oncol.* 2012;30(suppl):7522a.

9   Pao W, Miller VA, Politi KA, et al. Acquired resistance of lung adenocarcinomas to gefitinib or erlotinib is associated with a second mutation in the EGFR kinase domain. *PLoS Med.* 2005;2:e73.

10  Kobayashi S, Boggon TJ, Dayaram T, et al. EGFR mutation and resistance of non-small-cell lung cancer to gefitinib. *N Engl J Med.* 2005;352:786-792.

11  Kwak EL, Sordella R, Bell DW, et al. Irreversible inhibitors of the EGF receptor may circumvent acquired resistance to gefitinib. *Proc Natl Acad Sci U S A.* 2005;102:7665-7670.

12  Mok TS, Wu YL, Thongprasert S, et al. Gefitinib or carboplatin-paclitaxel in pulmonary adenocarcinoma. *N Engl J Med.* 2009;361:947-957.

13  Yun CH, Mengwasser KE, Toms AV, et al. The T790M mutation in EGFR kinase causes drug resistance by increasing the affinity for ATP. *Proc Natl Acad Sci U S A.* 2008;105:2070-2075.

14  Inukai M, Toyooka S, Ito S, et al. Presence of epidermal growth factor receptor gene T790M mutation as a minor clone in non-small cell lung cancer. *Cancer Res.* 2006;66:7854-7858.

15  Sequist LV, Martins RG, Spigel D, et al. First-line gefitinib in patients with advanced non-small-cell lung cancer harboring somatic EGFR mutations. *J Clin Oncol.* 2008;26:2442-2449.

16  Maheswaran S, Sequist LV, Nagrath S, et al. Detection of mutations in EGFR in circulating lung-cancer cells. *N Engl J Med.* 2008;359:366-377.

17  Girard N, Lou E, Azzoli CG, et al. Analysis of genetic variants in never-smokers with lung cancer facilitated by an Internet-based blood collection protocol: a preliminary report. *Clin Cancer Res.* 2010;16:755-763.

18  Shigematsu H, Lin L, Takahashi T, et al. Clinical and biological features associated with epidermal growth factor receptor gene mutations in lung cancers. *J Natl Cancer Inst.* 2005;97:339-346.

19  Kim YT, Kim TY, Lee DS, et al. Molecular changes of epidermal growth factor receptor (EGFR) and KRAS and their impact on the clinical outcomes in surgically resected adenocarcinoma of the lung. *Lung Cancer.* 2008;59:111-118.

**20**   Kosaka T, Yatabe Y, Onozato R, et al. Prognostic implication of EGFR, KRAS, and TP53 gene mutations in a large cohort of Japanese patients with surgically treated lung adenocarcinoma. *J Thorac Oncol.* 2009;4:22-29.

**21**   Lin CC, Hsu HH, Sun CT, et al. Chemotherapy response in East Asian non-small cell lung cancer patients harboring wild-type or activating mutation of epidermal growth factor receptors. *J Thorac Oncol.* 2010;5:1424-1429.

**22**   Cappuzzo F, Ligorio C, Toschi L, et al. EGFR and HER2 gene copy number and response to first-line chemotherapy in patients with advanced non-small cell lung cancer (NSCLC). *J Thorac Oncol.* 2007;2:423-429.

**23**   Tsao MS, Sakurada A, Ding K, et al. Prognostic and predictive value of epidermal growth factor receptor tyrosine kinase domain mutation status and gene copy number for adjuvant chemotherapy in non-small cell lung cancer. *J Thorac Oncol.* 2011;6:139-147.

**24**   Kim ES, Hirsh V, Mok T, et al. Gefitinib versus docetaxel in previously treated non-small-cell lung cancer (INTEREST): a randomised phase III trial. *Lancet.* 2008;372:1809-1818.

# Chapter 5

# EGFR-targeted therapies in non-small cell lung cancer

There are several possible strategies to achieve epidermal growth factor receptor (EGFR) pathway blockade, including different classes of compounds. The main strategies included agents that target the extracellular domain of the receptor, such as monoclonal antibodies, or small molecules that interfere with the tyrosine kinase activity of the intracellular domain, such as tyrosine kinase inhibitors (TKIs).

## Anti-EGFR monoclonal antibodies

Monoclonal antibodies bind to the extracellular portion of the receptor, thus preventing the interaction of ligand with EGFR receptor and consequently inhibit EGFR activation and the downstream cascade. A number of different antibodies have been developed, including cetuximab, necitumumab, panitumumab, and matuzumab, and some of them have gained regulatory approval for use in *EGFR*-overexpressing colorectal cancer and head and neck tumors. Cetuximab, a human-murine chimeric anti-EGFR immunoglobulin G (IgG) monoclonal antibody, represents the most extensively investigated agent in NSCLC.

### Cetuximab

In preclinical studies, cetuximab inhibited the growth of lung cancer cell lines and mouse xenografts, particularly in combination with chemotherapy [1,2]. A number of phase I and II clinical trials showed

© Springer International Publishing Switzerland 2014
F. Cappuzzo, *Guide to Targeted Therapies: EGFR mutations in NSCLC*, DOI 10.1007/978-3-319-03059-3_5

that the drug is active and can be safely administered to patients with metastatic non-small cell lung cancer (NSCLC) either alone or, more notably, in association with chemotherapy, encouraging further investigation of combination regimens [3–6]. For example, the Southwest Oncology Group (SWOG) conducted a phase II trial (S0342) to compare a concurrent versus a sequential schedule of cetuximab [7]. In this study, 223 chemotherapy-naïve patients with advanced NSCLC were randomized to carboplatin–paclitaxel plus cetuximab versus carboplatin–paclitaxel followed by cetuximab. No difference in response rate and progression-free survival was observed, while a median survival of 11 months was reported in both arms, suggesting that adding cetuximab to chemotherapy could improve survival as compared to chemotherapy alone.

The benefit of a combination approach including cetuximab has been further reinforced in the Lung Cancer Cetuximab Study, where 86 untreated patients with EGFR-positive tumors assessed by immunohistochemistry (IHC) were randomized to cisplatin–vinorelbine versus the same regimen plus cetuximab [8]. Although the trial was not designed to formally compare the two arms of treatment, a 1-month improvement in survival was observed in favor of the cetuximab arm (8.3 versus 7.3 months), thus suggesting that cetuximab could improve the efficacy of cisplatin–vinorelbine. This hypothesis was further tested in the FLEX (First-Line ErbituX in lung cancer) trial, a randomized phase III study of cisplatin–vinorelbine with or without cetuximab performed in 1125 patients with *EGFR*-expressing NSCLC in the first-line setting [9]. Importantly, the addition of cetuximab to chemotherapy led to a significant, though marginal, survival improvement (11.3 versus 10 months, hazard ratio [HR] 0.87, $P=0.044$) with an increased risk of adverse events, particularly febrile neutropenia. Similar results were observed in the BMS099 trial, a phase III trial that randomly assigned 676 chemotherapy-naïve patients with NSCLC to carboplatin plus a taxane versus the same chemotherapy regimen plus cetuximab [10]. Notably, patients were enrolled into the study regardless of *EGFR* expression. Although the primary endpoint of progression-free survival favoring the cetuximab arm was not met (4.4 versus 4.2 months; $P=0.2$), a non-significant trend toward longer survival (9.6 versus 8.3 months, HR 0.89, 95% CI 0.75–1.05, $P=0.17$)

was reported. Regulatory authorities considered these data not sufficient for recommending approval, judging the survival benefit and risks as disproportional.

The survival results observed in the FLEX and BMS099 trials clearly indicated that there is a consistent fraction of patients with NSCLC deriving no or little benefit from cetuximab therapy, thus highlighting the importance of proper patient selection. The presence of *EGFR* mutations, a critical factor for response to EGFR-TKIs, does not seem to be relevant for cetuximab sensitivity [11], as illustrated in Figure 5.1. Data in colorectal cancer (CRC) showed that increased *EGFR* gene copy number as detected by fluorescence in situ hybridization (FISH) might be associated with increased sensitivity to cetuximab, at least in terms of response and time to progression (TTP) [12,13]. In lung cancer, Hirsch et al analyzed the impact of *EGFR* gene copy number detected by FISH on survival of patients with NSCLC enrolled into the S0342 trial [14,15]. In this analysis [15], progression-free survival and survival were significantly longer in *EGFR FISH*-positive patients treated with cetuximab and chemotherapy than in *EGFR FISH*-negative patients receiving the same treatment (progression-free survival: 6 versus 3 months, $P=0.0008$; median survival: 15 versus 7 months, $P=0.04$). Khambata-Ford et al presented an extensive biomarker analysis conducted among individuals participating to the BMS099 trial [16]. In this study, no difference in progression-free survival was observed in the *FISH*-positive group irrespective of the treatment. Surprisingly, median survival was significantly longer among *EGFR FISH*-positive patients treated with chemotherapy alone versus *EGFR FISH*-positive patients treated with chemotherapy plus cetuximab (12.5 versus 8.6 months, $P=0.03$).

In CRC, the biomarker most useful for identifying those patients suitable for cetuximab therapy is *KRAS*; patients with metastatic CRC who harbor a *KRAS* mutation derive no benefit from cetuximab and *KRAS* testing is now used in clinical practice for guiding treatment selection [17]. In contrast, in the analysis conducted by Kambata-Ford in the BMS099 study [16], patients with *KRAS* mutation treated with cetuximab and chemotherapy had longer progression-free survival (5.6 versus 2.8 months) and longer survival (16.8 versus 10.8 months) than individuals treated

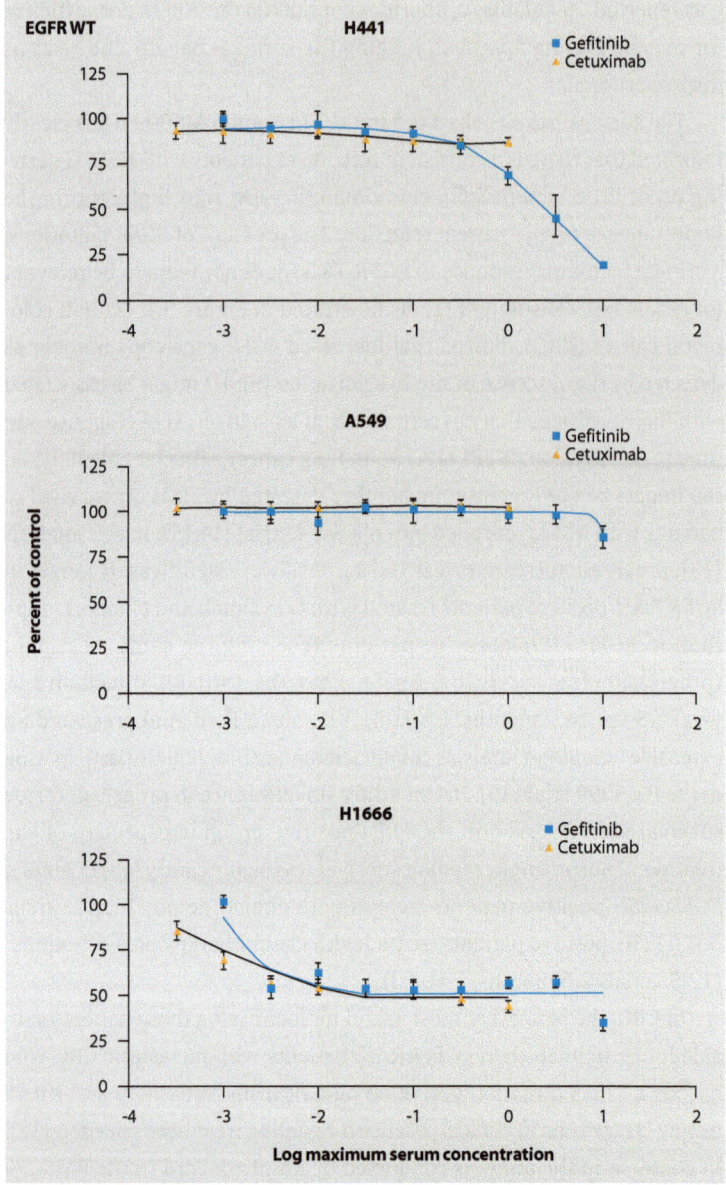

**Figure 5.1 Different effect of cetuximab and gefitinib in NSCLC cell-lines with or without *EGFR* mutations (continues opposite).**

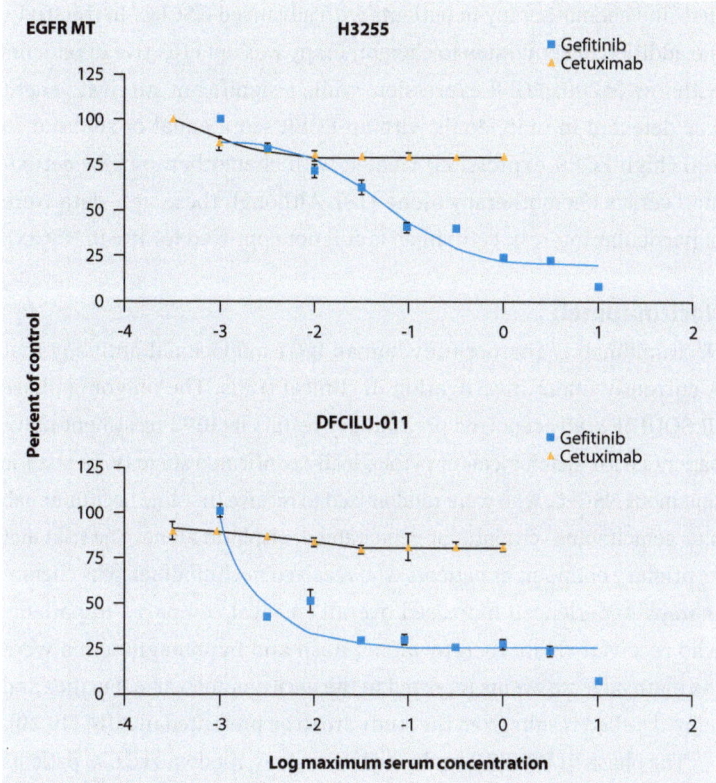

**Figure 5.1 Different effect of cetuximab and gefitinib in NSCLC cell-lines with or without** *EGFR* **mutations (continued).** The efficacy of gefitinib and cetuximab is different in cell lines with or without *EGFR* mutations. Presence of *EGFR* mutations is not critical for cetuximab sensitivity. MT, molecular therapy; WT, wild type. Reproduced with permission from © Oxford University Press 2014, Mukohara T et al [11].

with chemotherapy alone, even if the difference was not statistically significant (progression-free survival: $P=0.3$; survival: $P=0.93$). These findings suggest that *KRAS* mutations have different effects in advanced NSCLC and metastatic CRC, although the biologic reasons for this divergence are not completely understood.

More recently, Pirker et al re-analyzed the outcome of patients enrolled onto the FLEX trial, according to EGFR expression. By using a semi-quantitative method, the investigators demonstrated that high EGFR expression predicted survival benefit from the addition of cetuximab to first-line chemotherapy in patients with advanced NSCLC. In the study, the addition of cetuximab to chemotherapy was not effective in patients with low (<200) EGFR expression, while a significant survival benefit was detected in individuals with an EGFR score equal or superior to 200 (high EGFR expression) treated with chemotherapy plus cetuximab versus chemotherapy alone [18]. Although these new data were of particular interest, cetuximab is still not approved for use in NSCLC.

## Necitumumab

Necitumumab is another fully human IgG1 monoclonal antibody that is currently under investigation in clinical trials. The on-going phase III SQUIRE study reported preliminary results in 1093 treatment-naïve patients with histological- or cytologically-confirmed stage IV metastatic squamous NSCLC, who were randomized to receive first-line necitumumab plus gemcitabine–cisplatin or gemcitabine–cisplatin alone. The trial met its primary endpoint as patients who received necitumumab plus chemotherapy experienced increased overall survival compared to patients who received chemotherapy alone. Rash and hypomagnesemia were the main adverse events reported in the necitumumab arm. Further and more detailed results from the study are to be presented in 2014 [19,20].

The phase III INSPIRE study, led by Paz-Ares, randomized 633 patients with stage IV non-squamous NSCLC to necitumumab plus cisplatin–pemetrexed or cisplatin–pemetrexed alone. The necitumumab plus chemotherapy arm showed no benefit in overall survival (HR 1.01; $P=0.956$) or progression-free survival (HR 0.96; $P=0.664$), and due to adverse events it was recommended to stop enrollment into the study and discontinue necitumumab therapy, primarily due to fatal thromboembolic events that mostly occurred in the first two cycles of the study [21].

## EGFR tyrosine kinase inhibitors

Several compounds that reversibly or irreversibly bind to the EGFR tyrosine kinase domain have been developed, including gefitinib, erlotinib, and afatinib, which are now available in many countries for patients with NSCLC; Figure 5.2 demonstrates the mechanism of action of TKIs. Gefitinib and afatinib are approved for patients with *EGFR* mutations

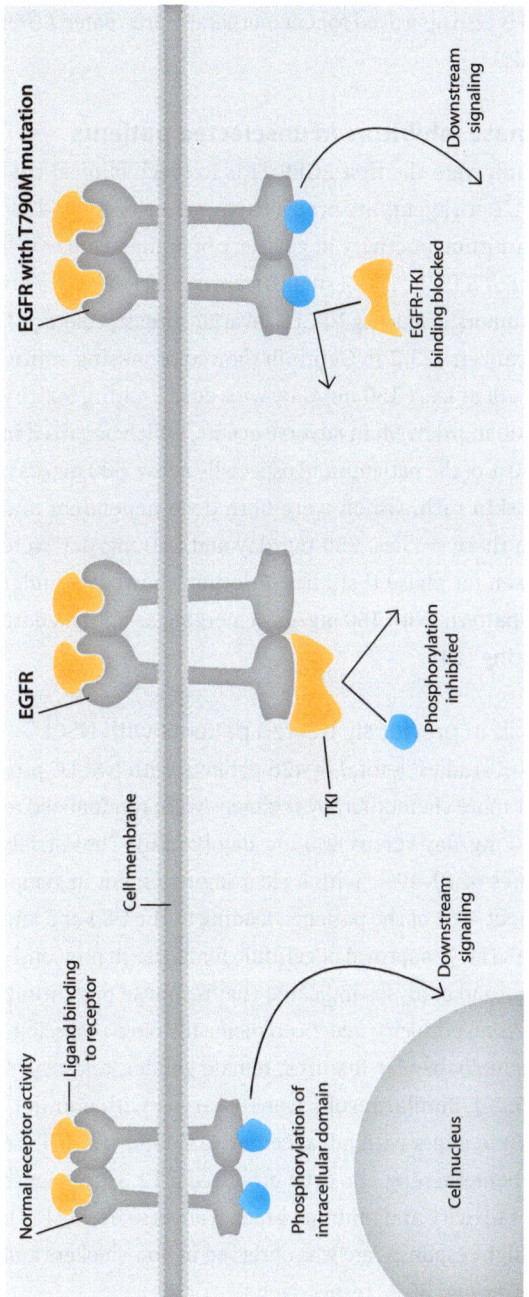

**Figure 5.2 Mechanism of action of EGFR tyrosine kinase inhibitors.** TKI, tyrosine kinase inhibitors.

only, while erlotinib is also approved for chemotherapy pretreated *EGFR* wild-type individuals.

## EGFR tyrosine kinase inhibitors in unselected patients

Gefitinib and erlotinib were the first EGFR-TKIs to reach clinical trial testing and approval. Both agents are orally active, selective EGFR-TKIs that demonstrated antitumor activity in a variety of human cancer cell lines overexpressing *EGFR* [22]. Phase I studies were conducted in patients with different solid tumors, including NSCLC, ovarian, breast, colorectal, and head and neck cancers [23,24]. Gefitinib showed promising antitumor activity at doses of at least 150 mg/day, with dose limiting toxicity observed at 800–1000 mg/day. Main adverse events, which occurred in approximately 70–80% of the patients and especially above 600 mg/day, were diarrhea and skin rash, which were both dose-dependent and reversible. Based on these studies, 250 mg/day and 500 mg/day were the fixed doses chosen for phase II studies. Erlotinib showed a similar activity and toxicity pattern, with 150 mg/day emerging as optimal dose for phase II trial testing [24].

### Gefitinib or erlotinib in previously treated patients with NSCLC

In the IDEAL-1 and -2 studies, a total of 426 patients with NSCLC progressing after one or more chemotherapy regimens were randomized to receive gefitinib 250 mg/day versus 500 mg/day [25,26]. These trials showed response rates of 10–19%, with a clear improvement in symptoms observed in about 40% of the patients, leading to the US Food and Drug Administration's (FDA) approval of gefitinib for its use in previously treated NSCLC. Subgroup analyses indicated that response to gefitinib was associated with Asian ethnicity, adenocarcinoma histology, especially in presence of bronchioloalveolar features, female gender, and never-smoking history [25,26]. Similar results were observed with erlotinib. In a phase II study in patients with advanced NSCLC following failure of platinum based chemotherapy, the drug produced a 12.3% response rate, with no grade 4 toxicity and minimal grade 3 adverse events [27]. As with gefitinib, a high response rate was observed in non-smokers and adenocarcinomas (37% and 30%, respectively).

Two large randomized phase III studies assessed gefitinib and erlo-tinib monotherapy in patients with advanced NSCLC who had failed at least one chemotherapy regimen [28,29]. The ISEL trial included 1692 patients who were randomized to gefitinib 250 mg/day or placebo [28]. Despite a higher response rate and longer TTP in the gefitinib arm, the study concluded that the drug produced no survival advantage over best supportive care in patients with advanced NSCLC (5.6 versus 5.1 months, $P=0.09$). Conversely, the BR21 trial, in which 731 pretreated patients with advanced NSCLC were randomized to receive erlotinib 150 mg/day or placebo, succeeded in meeting its primary endpoint, with patients in the experimental arm experiencing a statistically significant improvement in overall survival (HR 0.70, 95% CI 0.58–0.85, $P<0.001$) [29]. Results from these large randomized trials led to the approval of erlotinib monotherapy by the FDA for the treatment of patients with previously treated NSCLC and to restrictions for gefitinib use, limiting administration of gefitinib to patients already receiving and benefiting from the agent, or patients who have previously received and benefited from gefitinib. In two other studies, the INTEREST (Iressa NSCLC Trial Evaluating REsponse and Survival versus Taxotere) and the V-15-32 trial, gefitinib had similar efficacy to docetaxel when used as second-line therapy in patients progressing after platinum-based chemotherapy [27,30]. In the Iressa® as Second-line Therapy in Advanced NSCLC–KoreA (ISTANA) study, second-line gefitinib significantly prolonged progression-free survival as compared with docetaxel in Korean patients [31]. Moreover, a meta-analysis [32] including data from four randomized trials [27,30,31,33] confirmed that gefitinib had similar efficacy to that of docetaxel in unselected, pretreated patients with NSCLC. More recently, two randomized studies and a meta-analysis showed superiority of doc-etaxel versus erlotinib in patients with NSCLC lacking EGFR mutations [34–36]. In the TArceva Italian Lung Optimization tRial (TAILOR) study, a total of 220 EGFR wild-type patients were randomized to erlotinib or docetaxel second-line [34]. Although response rate and progression-free survival significantly favored the docetaxel arm, no difference in survival was detected. Okan et al randomly assigned 300 unselected patients with NSCLC to a second-line therapy with erlotinib or docetaxel

[35]. The study did not show any survival difference between the two treatments, even if a significant improvement in progression-free survival favored EGFR wild-type patients treated with docetaxel. Finally, a recent meta-analysis showed that second- or third-line EGFR-TKIs are inferior to chemotherapy in terms of progression-free survival but not in terms of overall survival [36].

## Gefitinib or erlotinib as first-line therapy

Four large prospective studies (INTACT 1 and 2, TRIBUTE, TALENT), including more than 4000 patients with advanced NSCLC, randomly assigned untreated patients to standard chemotherapy plus a TKI, or the same chemotherapy regimen plus placebo [37–40]. All trials failed to demonstrate any survival advantage for patients receiving the TKI, probably because of the lack of patient selection. Additional studies investigated the efficacy of gefitinib or erlotinib in previously untreated patients not selected for any biological characteristic. Phase II studies in unselected patients with NSCLC suggested that gefitinib or erlotinib are less effective than standard platinum-based chemotherapy as front-line setting in terms of response rate and progression-free survival, but with comparable survival [41–46], as illustrated in Table 5.1. These data suggested that front-line EGFR-TKI therapy in unselected patients could be a potential option because, even if the EGFR-TKI was less effective than chemotherapy, no detrimental effect on survival was observed. Based on this hypothesis, Italian investigators evaluated the possibility of giving erlotinib as a front-line therapy in unselected patients with NSCLC [47]. In the Tarceva® Or Chemotherapy (TORCH) study, 760 patients with NSCLC were randomly assigned to a standard therapy of chemotherapy followed by erlotinib at the time of progression versus the experimental arm of erlotinib first-line followed by chemotherapy at the time of progression. The study was discontinued when an interim analysis revealed that first-line erlotinib was inferior in unselected patients to the reverse, standard strategy of first-line cisplatin–gemcitabine followed by second-line erlotinib [47]. The Tarceva® Or Placebo In Clinically Advanced Lung cancer (TOPICAL) study showed that erlotinib did not significantly improve overall survival when added to best supportive care (as compared with

| Reference | # | Line | Drug | RR (%) | PFS (months) | OS (months) |
|---|---|---|---|---|---|---|
| Akerley | 41 | I | Erlotinib | 15 | 1.9 | 11.5 |
| Giaccone | 42 | I | Erlotinib | 22.7 | 2.7 | 12.8 |
| Niho | 43 | I | Gefitinib | 30 | NR | 13.9 |
| Hesketh | 44 | I | Erlotinib | 8 | 2.1 | 5 |
| Govindan | 45 | I | Gefitinib | 6.3 | NR | 6 |
| Jackman | 46 | I | Erlotinib | 10 | 3.5 | 10.9 |

**Table 5.1 Phase II data of EGFR-TKI efficacy in unselected patients with NSCLC.** Phase II trials showed that in unselected patients with NSCLC gefitinib or erlotinib seemed to produce similar survival to that previously observed with platinum-based chemotherapy. These data led to the hypothesis (later disproved) that an EGFR-TKI can be used front-line irrespective of *EGFR* status. OS, overall survival; PFS, progression-free survival; RR, response rate; TKI, tyrosine kinase inhibitors. Adapted from Akerley et al [41], Giaccone et al [42], Niho et al [43], Hesketh et al [44], Govindan et al [45], Jackman et al [46].

best supportive care alone) in a population of chemotherapy-naïve patients who had a poor performance status (Eastern Cooperative Oncology Group [ECOG] PS 2/3) or who were unfit for platinum chemotherapy; however, there was a trend for a prolongation of progression-free survival and a significant prolongation of both overall survival and progression-free survival in the subset of female patients [48]. In the Iressa® in NSCLC versus vinorelbine investigation in the elderly (INVITE) study, 196 elderly and biologically unselected patients with NSCLC were randomly assigned to front-line therapy with vinorelbine or gefitinib [49]. The study, designed for demonstrating a superiority of gefitinib versus vinorelbine in terms of progression-free survival, failed to demonstrate any difference between the two treatments. Overall, these data clearly demonstrated that EGFR-TKIs are not effective as front-line therapy in unselected patients with NSCLC.

## Gefitinib or erlotinib as maintenance therapy

Significant improvements in progression-free survival have been observed with EGFR-TKI maintenance therapy following platinum-based chemotherapy in unselected patients [50–54]. In the SATURN trial, patients with NSCLC not progressing after four cycles of platinum-based chemotherapy were randomized to erlotinib or placebo [50]. The study met its primary and secondary endpoints, showing that patients receiving erlotinib had a significant reduction in the risk of progression

(HR 0.71, 95% CI 0.62–0.82, $P<0.0001$) and death (HR 0.81, 95% CI 0.70–0.95, $P=0.0088$). The greatest progression-free survival benefit was observed in patients with *EGFR* mutations, although a progression-free survival improvement was also detected in the *EGFR* wild-type population. Interestingly, overall survival was significantly prolonged in the known *EGFR* wild-type population, but not in the known *EGFR* mutation positive population. In the Avastin Tarceva Lung Adenocarcinoma Study (ATLAS), patients with metastatic NSCLC not progressing after four cycles of platinum-based chemotherapy plus bevacizumab were randomly assigned to bevacizumab plus placebo or erlotinib [51]. The results of the ATLAS trial confirmed that the addition of erlotinib significantly reduced the risk of progression (HR 0.71, 95% CI 0.58–0.86, $P<0.001$), with the highest benefit observed in the *EGFR* mutated population. No statistically significant overall survival differences were observed in the ATLAS study in either the overall population (HR 0.92, 95% CI 0.70–1.21, $P=0.53$), or known *EGFR* mutant (HR 0.46, 95% CI 0.21–1.02) or wild-type patients (HR 0.86, 95% CI 0.65–1.15).

Due to its efficacy in advanced pretreated patients with NSCLC and its mild toxicity profile, gefitinib has also been investigated as a maintenance therapy. In unselected patients, two studies evaluating the efficacy of gefitinib as maintenance therapy after three cycles of platinum-based chemotherapy in patients with metastatic disease or after chemoradiation in patients with locally advanced disease failed to demonstrate any beneficial effect of the experimental treatment [52,53]. Nevertheless, a subgroup analysis of one of the studies showed that maintenance gefitinib significantly improved survival in the patients with adenocarcinoma [52]. More recently, Zhang et al [54] reported the final results of the INFORM (Iressa in NSCLC FOR Maintenance, C-TONG0804) trial, a phase III study of gefitinib versus placebo as maintenance treatment in Chinese patients with molecularly unselected locally advanced or metastatic NSCLC who had achieve disease control after completion of four cycles of platinum-based doublet chemotherapy. Patients treated with gefitinib had a 58% relative reduction in risk of progression compared with those receiving placebo (4.8 versus 2.6 months; HR 0.42, 95% CI 0.33–0.55, $P<0.0001$), while overall survival did not differ between the two groups (median survival 18.7 versus 16.9 months; HR 0.84, 95% CI 0.62–1.14, $P$=0.26). Sequential anti-EGFR therapy was also associated with higher disease control rate (72% versus 51%, $P$=0.0001) and better symptom control. Although tissue collection was not mandatory for study entry, 79 patients (27%) provided tumor tissue for EGFR status assessment and activating mutations were found in 30 samples (38%). Compared to the intention to treat population, in *EGFR* mutant patients the improvement in progression-free survival was greater (16.6 versus 2.8 months; HR 0.17, 95% CI 0.07–0.42, $P$<0.0001) with no evidence of benefit in the *EGFR* wild-type population. INFORM data confirmed again that *EGFR* mutations are the best predictor of response to an EGFR-TKI and consequently *EGFR* mutant patients gain the greater benefit when treated early during the course of their disease. Moreover, it is confirmed that Asian patients have a higher incidence of hidden *EGFR* mutations.

## Afatinib in previously treated NSCLC

Afatinib is an orally available, irreversible EGFR, HER2, and HER4 inhibitor that has shown preclinical activity against cancer cells harboring common activating *EGFR* mutations and the *T790M* mutation, albeit with a lower potency [55]. By irreversibly and covalently binding to the ATP-binding site in the kinase domains of EGFR and HER, afatinib suppresses receptor kinase activity longer than reversible EGFR-TKIs. Additionally, the irreversible binding of afatinib to HER2 deactivates the dimerization partner of EGFR, which stops the dimer formation that stimulates the receptors' tyrosine kinase activity [56]. Phase I studies established the maximum tolerated dose at 50 mg/day orally, with diarrhea and rash as most common adverse events [57]. Afatinib was evaluated in a large phase III study in patients with acquired resistance to erlotinib or gefitinib. The LUX-LUNG 1 trial [58] randomly allocated 585 patients with NSCLC to afatinib 50 mg/day or placebo. Eligible patients had received one or two previous chemotherapy regimens and had disease progression after at least 12 weeks of treatment with erlotinib or gefitinib. Patients were not selected based on *EGFR* mutation status. The median overall survival (primary endpoint) in the two arms was not different, although a significant difference in progression-free survival was observed

(3.3 versus 1.1 months, $P<0.0001$ by independent review). Once again, the negative results of this study highlighted the relevance of a patient selection based on tumor biology.

## EGFR tyrosine kinase inhibitors in patients harboring activating *EGFR* mutations

Several phase II and III studies have evaluated the efficacy of gefitinib, erlotinib, or afatinib in patients harboring classical (exon 19 deletion or L858 substitutions in exon 21) *EGFR* mutations. Table 5.2 illustrates results from phase III trials comparing an EGFR-TKI versus platinum-based chemotherapy in untreated patients harboring *EGFR* mutations [59–66]. At the present time, no phase III study has directly compared these three EGFR-TKIs and, therefore, it is not possible to determine if there is any difference in their efficacy or toxicity. Based on this author's experience, indirect comparisons suggest that gefitinib and erlotinib are better tolerated than afatinib, with no difference in terms of response rate and with a potential superiority of afatinib in terms of progression-free survival.

### Studies with gefitinib

Several phase II trials have investigated the efficacy of gefitinib as a first-line treatment in selected patient populations, based on the presence of activating *EGFR* gene mutations [67–76]. In a phase II trial in this setting, Asahina and colleagues observed a response rate of 75% and median progression-free survival of 8.9 months [67] and Yang et al reported an impressive 95% response rate in a cohort of 43 patients with exon 19 deletion or L858R mutations [69]. Sequist et al [70] selected 98 chemotherapy-naïve patients with non-squamous histology who had at least one clinical characteristic associated with activating *EGFR* mutations (low or never smoking history, adenocarcinoma histology, female gender, and East Asian ethnicity). In this clinically enriched patient population, 34 patients (35%) had *EGFR* mutations and 31 received gefitinib treatment. The overall response rate was 55% and median progression-free survival was 9.2 months. Because of the favorable toxicity profile, Inoue et al evaluated gefitinib in a phase II trial in patients with NSCLC with a poor performance status of 3 and 4, who harbored *EGFR* mutations, and

| Study | EGFR TKI | n | Median PFS in TKI arm (months) | P value | HR |
|---|---|---|---|---|---|
| First signal | Gefitinib | 42 | 8.4 | 0.084 | 0.61 |
| IPASS | Gefitinib | 261 | 9.5 | <0.0001 | 0.48 |
| WJTOG 3405 | Gefitinib | 177 | 9.2 | <0.001 | 0.48 |
| NEJSG 002 | Gefitinib | 200 | 10.8 | <0.001 | 0.36 |
| OPTIMAL | Erlotinib | 154 | 13.1 | <0.0001 | 0.16 |
| EURTAC | Erlotinib | 174 | 9.7 | 0.0001 | 0.37 |
| LUX-3 | Afatinib | 345 | 11.1 | 0.001 | 0.58 |
| LUX-6 | Afatinib | 364 | 11.0 | <0.0001 | 0.28 |

**Table 5.2 Studies of EGFR tyrosine kinase inhibitors versus chemotherapy as first-line therapy in patients with *EGFR* mutated NSCLC**. PFS, progression-free survival; TKI, tyrosine kinase inhibitor. Adapted from Han et al [59], Mok et al [60], Mitsudomi et al [61], Maemondo et al [62], Zhou et al [63], Rosell et al [64], Sequist et al [65], Wu et al [66].

who were not eligible for chemotherapy [71]. The impressive 66% response rate observed, along with a median overall survival of 17.8 months, in an unfavorable subset of NSCLC indicated that all patients with *EGFR* mutations should be treated with EGFR-TKIs, including those with very poor performance status.

Four phase III studies (IPASS, First-SIGNAL, WJTOG3405, and NEJ002) compared gefitinib versus chemotherapy as first-line therapy in patients with *EGFR* mutations or with clinical characteristics predictive for the presence of *EGFR* mutations [59–62]. The IPASS trial was a randomized phase III study where previously untreated patients in East Asia who had advanced lung adenocarcinoma and who were non-smokers or former light smokers were randomized to receive gefitinib or carboplatin–paclitaxel [60]. The primary objective was to assess the non-inferiority of gefitinib versus carboplatin–paclitaxel for progression-free survival. The study exceeded the primary objective, demonstrating the superiority of gefitinib over chemotherapy in terms of progression-free survival in the intent-to-treat population (HR 0.74, 95% CI 0.65–0.85, $P<0.001$). No difference in overall survival was observed, probably because of the confounding effect of post-study treatments, particularly exposure to gefitinib or other

EGFR-TKIs. Importantly, the progression-free survival benefit observed in this trial was confined to patients harboring *EGFR* mutations, with a clear detrimental effect of gefitinib in *EGFR* wild-type individuals. From a clinical point of view, two very relevant findings derived from this work: first, an EGFR-TKI can be used as a front-line therapy only in patients with activating *EGFR* mutations; second, the presence of certain clinical characteristics is not sufficient for proper patient selection.

Another trial compared gefitinib with cisplatin–gemcitabine as first-line treatment in Asian never-smokers, with advanced adenocarcinoma [59]. Three hundred and nine patients, mostly women (89%), were randomly allocated 1:1 to gefitinib 250 mg/day or cisplatin–gemcitabine. The primary endpoint was overall survival. In the whole population, no difference in response, progression-free survival, or overall survival was detected. Nevertheless, when the analysis was restricted to patients harboring *EGFR* mutations, similarly to the IPASS study, response rate and progression-free survival were significantly in favor of gefitinib, with no difference in terms of survival, most likely due to the post-study use of EGFR-TKIs in 80.7% of subjects enrolled in the chemotherapy arm. The results of this study confirmed that clinical characteristics alone cannot be used in clinical practice for selecting patients eligible for first-line EGFR-TKIs.

Two phase III Japanese studies have been performed specifically in patients with *EGFR* mutations to compare the efficacy of gefitinib versus chemotherapy in the first-line treatment of NSCLC [61,62]. In the WJTOG3405 trial, 172 patients with *EGFR* mutations were randomly assigned to receive gefitinib or chemotherapy with cisplatin–docetaxel [61]. The study met its primary endpoint, showing a median progression-free survival of 9.2 months in the gefitinib group and 6.3 months in the chemotherapy group. Finally, the NEJ002 trial randomly assigned patients with NSCLC harboring *EGFR* mutations to gefitinib or chemotherapy with carboplatin and paclitaxel [62]. The study confirmed that gefitinib was superior to chemotherapy in terms of progression-free survival (10.4 versus 5.5 months), reinforcing the evidence that EGFR-TKIs should be preferred to chemotherapy in presence of *EGFR* mutations.

The TheraScreen®: EGFR29 Mutation Kit (QIAGEN Group, Venlo, Netherlands) is CE-in vitro diagnostic (IVD)-marked real-time PCR assay.

TheraScreen acts as a companion diagnostic test for gefitinib and afatinib by combining the ARMS and Scorpion fluorescent primer/probe systems to detect 29 mutations in exons 18, 19, 20, and 21 of the *EGFR* gene.

## Studies with erlotinib

The efficacy of erlotinib versus standard platinum-based chemotherapy in untreated patients with activating *EGFR* mutations has been evaluated in two large phase III studies [63,64]. In 2011, Zhou and colleagues published the results of the OPTIMAL trial, a phase III study comparing erlotinib to carboplatin–gemcitabine in Chinese patients harboring *EGFR* mutations [63]. A striking HR of 0.16 (95% CI 0.10–0.26) for progression-free survival was reported for subjects receiving the experimental treatment (median progression-free survival: 13.1 months versus 4.6 months for erlotinib and standard chemotherapy, respectively). The enormous difference between the two arms was related to the unexpected low performance of the chemotherapy arm (Figure 5.3). Moreover, the OPTIMAL trial was conducted on Chinese patients, raising the question whether a similar difference in outcome could be observed in Caucasians. In 2009, Rosell and the Spanish Lung Cancer Group published the results of a prospective trial evaluating the feasibility of a large-scale screening program

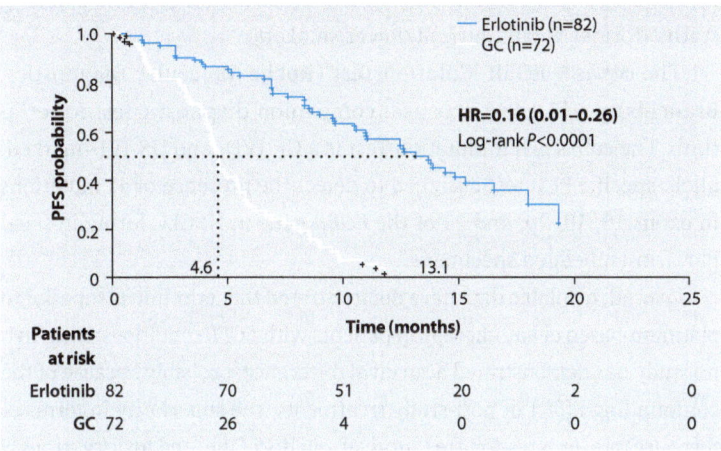

**Figure 5.3 Progression-free survival in the OPTIMAL trial: erlotinib versus chemotherapy.**
GC, gemcitabine–carboplatin; PFS, progression-free survival. Reproduced with permission from © Elsevier Limited 2014, Zhou et al [63].

for detecting *EGFR* mutations in patients with metastatic NSCLC [77]. Patients with proven *EGFR* mutations were then considered for erlotinib in any line of treatment. More than 2100 subjects from 129 institutes were prospectively tested. *EGFR* mutations were detected in 350 patients (16%), above all women, never smokers, and patients with adenocarcinoma. Two hundred and seventeen patients received erlotinib as first-line (113 patients) or second–third-line treatment (104 patients). Median progression-free survival was 14 months, similar to that reported in Asian populations. The same group coordinated a large phase III study (EURTAC) comparing, for the first time in Caucasian chemotherapy-naïve patients with *EGFR* mutations, erlotinib versus standard platinum-based chemotherapy [64]. The study met its primary endpoint of progression-free survival; patients receiving erlotinib had a 63% relative reduction in risk of progression compared with those receiving standard chemotherapy (9.7 months versus 5.2 months, HR 0.37, 95% CI 0.25–0.54, $P<0.0001$). A higher response rate (58% versus 15%, intention to treat population) and more favorable toxicity profile were associated with erlotinib. In the subgroup analyses a significant progression-free survival benefit favored erlotinib independently of age (>65 years versus <65 years), gender, performance status (ECOG PS 0 versus 1 versus 2), histology (adenocarcinoma versus other histology), and smoking status (former versus current/never smokers).

The cobas® EGFR Mutation Test (Roche Molecular Diagnostics, Branchburg, NJ, USA) acts as a companion diagnostic test for erlotinib. The cobas EGFR Mutation Test is a CE-IVD- and US-IVD-marked, allele-specific PCR test designed to detect the presence of 41 mutations in exons 18, 19, 20, and 21 of the *EGFR* gene in NSCLC formalin-fixed paraffin-embedded specimens.

Overall, available data have demonstrated that erlotinib is superior to platinum-based chemotherapy in patients with *EGFR* mutations. Although no study has demonstrated a survival difference, probably because of the confounding effect of post-study treatments, the superiority in terms of response rate, progression-free survival, quality of life, and toxicity strongly support erlotinib in first-line setting in *EGFR*-selected patients with NSCLC.

## Studies with afatinib

The role of the irreversible EGFR-TKI afatinib in the first-line setting in patients harboring *EGFR* mutations has been investigated in three studies. The first, the LUX-LUNG 2, was a phase II trial exploring the efficacy of afatinib in patients with stage IIIb/IV, *EGFR* mutated NSCLC [78]. The study, enrolling patients untreated or previously exposed to chemotherapy, was subsequently amended to allow only untreated patients. The primary endpoint was objective response rate by independent radiologic review. Among the 129 enrolled patients, 61 received afatinib as first-line treatment and 68 received it as second-line treatment, 99 received 50 mg/day orally as starting dose and 30 received 40 mg/day orally. One hundred and six patients presented the common exon 19 or 21 *EGFR* mutations and 23 patients presented with the other less common mutations. The objective response rate in the overall population was 61% by independent review and 60% by investigator assessment, while the objective response rate by independent review in common and uncommon mutations subgroups was 66% and 39%, respectively. Drug-related adverse events, mainly diarrhea and skin rash, were observed in the vast majority of cases, with about a quarter of patients experiencing grade 3 adverse events with the 50 mg dose, thus suggesting that the daily dose of 40 mg could be preferable for additional studies.

Two phase III trials have subsequently investigated afatinib in the front-line, *EGFR* mutation-positive setting. The LUX-LUNG 3 [65], a multicenter, randomized, open-label phase III study compared afatinib with cisplatin plus pemetrexed in patients with locally advanced or metastatic lung adenocarcinoma harboring *EGFR* mutations. Among the 1269 screened patients, 345 were eligible and were randomized in a two-to-one fashion to afatinib 40 mg/day or chemotherapy up to a maximum of six cycles and without any maintenance therapy. As expected, patients were mainly East Asian, never-smokers, and women. *EGFR* mutations were predominantly exon 19 deletions and L858R point mutations. The progression-free survival assessed by independent review, the primary endpoint of this trial, was significantly prolonged in the afatinib arm compared to chemotherapy arm, with median progression-free survival of 11.1 and 6.9 months, as illustrated in Figure 5.4; median

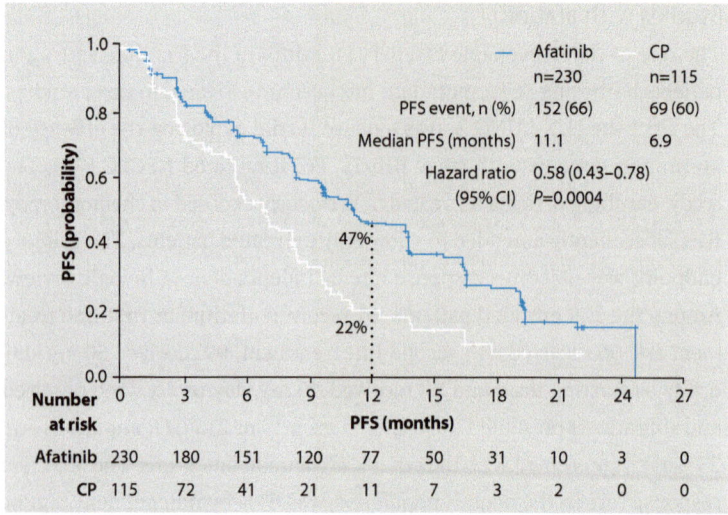

**Figure 5.4 Progression-free-survival in the LUX-LUNG 3 trial: afatinib versus chemotherapy.**
CP, cisplatin–pemetrexed; PFS, progression-free survival. Reproduced with permission from
© Yang JC-H, Schuler M, Yamamoto N, et al; on behalf of LUX-Lung 3 investigators. LUX-Lung 3:
a randomized, open-label, Phase III study of afatinib vs cisplatin/pemetrexed as 1st-line treatment
for patients with advanced adenocarcinoma of the lung harboring EGFR-activating mutations.
Slides presented at: 2012 ASCO Annual Meeting; June 1-June 5, 2013; Chicago, IL. Abstract
LBA7500 [79].

progression-free survival was 13.6 versus 6.9 months in patients with
classical (exon 19 deletion or exon 21) *EGFR* mutations.

Afatinib achieved a higher response rate compared with chemotherapy, according to both independent (56% versus 23%) and investigator
(69% versus 44%) assessment and higher disease control rate (90% versus
81% by independent review). The most frequent (≥20% incidence)
adverse reactions in the afatinib arm were diarrhea, rash/dermatitis
acneiform, stomatitis, paronychia, dry skin, decreased appetite, and
pruritus. Although grade ≥3 treatment-related adverse events occurred
in nearly 50% of patients receiving afatinib, the treatment was discontinued just in 8% of patients. Pre-dose plasma samples on days one and
eight of cycle two and day one of cycle three demonstrate that dose
modification, due to individual tolerability, optimized the exposure to
afatinib, holding efficacious plasma levels [80].

In the third study, LUX-LUNG 6 [66], Asian patients harboring *EGFR*
mutations were randomized 2:1 to receive afatinib 40 mg/day or cisplatin

plus gemcitabine. The study showed that patients treated with afatinib had a significantly longer progression-free survival than individuals receiving chemotherapy (median progression-free survival 11.0 versus 5.6 months, $P<0.0001$), as well as higher response rate (66.9% versus 23.0%, $P<0.0001$) and higher disease control rate (92.6% versus 60.2%, $P<0.0001$). Overall, afatinib data demonstrated that the drug is effective in patients with *EGFR* mutations, supporting its use in front-line setting.

As mentioned on page 46, the TheraScreen: EGFR29 Mutation Kit acts as a companion diagnostic test for afatinib and gefitinib. By combining the ARMS and Scorpion system, the kit can detect 29 mutations in exons 18, 19, 20, and 21 of the *EGFR* gene.

## Other irreversible inhibitors

Among new irreversible inhibitors, dacomitinib is one of the most promising agents. Dacomitinib is an irreversible EGFR, HER2, and HER4 inhibitor with a higher kinase inhibition than gefitinib/erlotinib in both gefitinib/erlotinib-sensitive and in *EGFR*-T790M- and *HER2*-mutated cell lines [81]. After a phase I trial, recruiting pretreated patients with NSCLC and establishing the maximum tolerated dose at 45 mg/day orally [82], a phase II study performed in patients with NSCLC after failure of ≥1 chemotherapy regimen and erlotinib showed a promising activity and a meaningful improvements in the patient-reported outcomes [83]. A large phase II study randomly assigned 188 pretreated patients with NSCLC to dacomitinib or erlotinib. In the overall population, progression-free survival, the primary endpoint of the study, was 12.4 weeks for dacomitinib arm and 8.3 weeks for erlotinib arm; the progression-free survival benefit was consistent across several subgroups and particularly remarkable in patients with *KRAS* wild-type tumors, with a median progression-free survival of 16.1 weeks versus 8.3 weeks in the experimental and control arm, respectively [84]. The phase III, multicenter, double-blinded ARCHER 1009 study compared dacomitinib to erlotinib in two co-primary populations of pretreated patients with advanced NSCLC (all enrolled patients and patients with KRAS wild-type mutations). The top-line results from ARCHER 1009 reported in January 2014 stated that dacomitinib did not significantly improve progression-free survival compared to erlotinib in either treatment group [85,86]. A recent study evaluated the efficacy of dacomitinib in front-line setting in patients with NSCLC with activating *EGFR* mutations. The study showed that dacomitinib is particularly effective with a response rate of 74% and a median progression-free survival of 16.8 months [87]. Based on these data, the ARCHER 1050, a phase III, open-label trial has been initiated to compare the efficacy of first-line dacomitinib versus gefitinib in 440 *EGFR* mutant patients with stage IIIB/IV NSCLC. The primary endpoint is progression-free survival by independent radiologic review. This trial is ongoing, with no data currently available [88].

## Different *EGFR* mutations, different sensitivity to EGFR tyrosine kinase inhibitors
### Uncommon mutations (other than T790M)

Although the presence of *EGFR* mutations predicts sensitivity to EGFR-TKIs, available data indicate that the type of mutation influences the efficacy of gefitinib, erlotinib, or afatinib (Figure 5.5) [60,61,63]. In the IPASS study, gefitinib achieved a higher tumor response rate against tumors with exon 19 mutations as compared with exon 21 deletions [50]. There are limited data suggesting that exon 19 deletions may predict a longer overall survival and/or progression-free survival after EGFR-TKI therapy than the L858R point mutation [46,89–91]. In a pooled analysis of five trials, patients with exon 19 deletions had a longer median TTP (14.6 versus 9.7 months; $P=0.02$) and overall survival (30.8 versus 14.8 months; $P<0.001$) than those with L858R mutations. However, the prospective, randomized WJTOG3405 and North East Japan Study Group trials did not find a significant difference in progression-free survival between patients with these mutations, regardless of the treatment arm [61,62]. A potential biological basis for a greater efficacy of EGFR-TKI against exon 19 mutated tumors is suggested by evidence that in untreated patients *EGFR* amplification occurs invariably in exon 19 mutants (rather than in wild-type or other mutants) and confers an advantage in these cells [92]. This suggests that exon 19 mutants may be particularly dependent on EGFR signaling and are thus especially sensitive to its inhibition by EGFR-TKI [61]. In addition, biochemical studies suggest that erlotinib is a much better inhibitor of EGFR in the presence of the exon 19 deletion compared to L858R, which may also contribute to the clinical observations [93].

In addition to the classical mutations in exon 19 (deletion) and 21 (L858R), several other *EGFR* mutations have been reported. In clinical practice, detection of a rare *EGFR* mutation in a chemotherapy-naïve patient raises the question as to whether a front-line therapy with EGFR-TKIs is appropriate or whether standard chemotherapy should be preferable. Few data are available on the predictive role of uncommon *EGFR* mutations. Some *EGFR* mutations are certainly associated with sensitivity to gefitinib, erlotinib, or afatinib, including the Gly719 on exon 18 and Leu861 on exon 21. In 2007, Mitsudomi reported a response rate to EGFR-TKIs of 55.6% for G719 mutation [94]. In another study, Wu and colleagues analyzed 627 *EGFR* mutant patients and found 15 G719 mutations and 15 L861 mutations. All subjects had received a TKI treatment, with a response rate of 53.3% for G719 and of 60% for L861 [95].

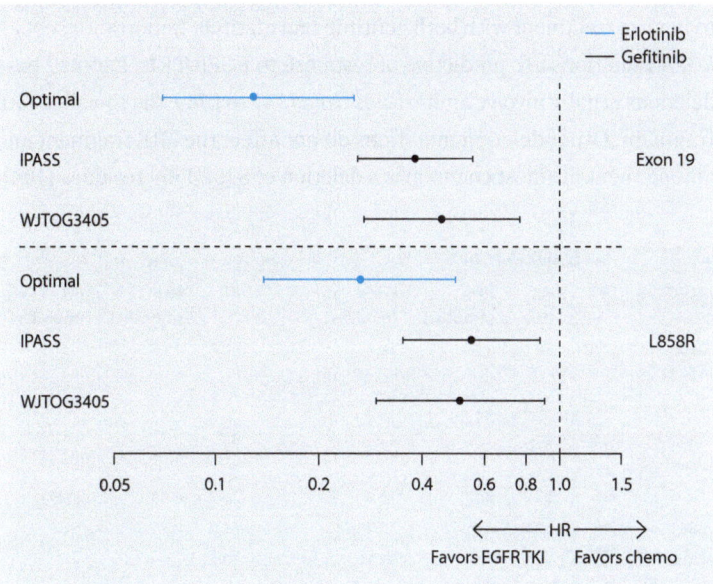

**Figure 5.5 Type of *EGFR* mutation and effect of progression-free survival in randomized phase III studies, comparing EGFR tyrosine kinase inhibitors versus chemotherapy.**
TKI, tyrosine kinases inhibitors. Adapted from Mok et al [56], Mitsudomi et al [61], Zhou et al [63].

Recently, Yang et al analyzed the outcome of patients enrolled in three clinical trials with afatinib (LUX-LUNG 2, 3, 6), according to presence of *EGFR* uncommon mutations [96]. In this study, the G719 mutation was detected in 18 cases and the L861 in 16 cases. Response rate to afatinib was 78% for the G719 mutation and 56% for the L861 mutation. Therefore, patients harboring the G719 or the L861 mutations are sensitive to EGFR-TKIs and it is reasonable to offer such agents as first-line therapy (Table 5.3).

Several aberrations in exon 19 have been described in NSCLC, both deletions and insertions. Exon 19 insertion mutations have been described in 0.2% of patients with NSCLC and represent about 1% of all *EGFR* mutations [100]. Insertions in exon 19 usually result in the substitution of a proline for a leucine at residue 747. The few clinical data available [101–103] suggested that such mutations could also be predictive for EGFR-TKI response. In the He et al study, investigators cloned the full-length *EGFR* gene and transfected Ba/F3 and NIH-3T3 cell lines, demonstrating that *EGFR* exon 19 insertions are oncogenic and that transformed cell lines are sensitive to in vitro treatment with both gefitinib and afatinib. Importantly, not all *EGFR* mutations are predictive of response to EGFR-TKIs. Exon 19 base deletions usually involve amino acids from L747 to E749, the so-called LRE fragment. Other deletion mutations do not affect the LRE fragment and among them the most common is a deletion of S752-I769 residues [104].

| EGRF | Reversible EGFR-TKIs | | | | Afatinib | | | |
|---|---|---|---|---|---|---|---|---|
| | N | RR (%) | PFS (months) | OS (months) | N | RR (%) | PFS (months) | OS (months) |
| Exon 19–21 | 278 | 74.1 | 8.5 | 19.6 | 308 | 60.8 | 13.6 | – |
| Wild-type | 272 | 16.5 | 2.0 | 10.4 | 42 | 0 | 1.0 | 7.2 |
| Exon 20 insertion | 11 | 0 | 1.4 | 4.8 | 20 | 8.7 | 2.7 | 9.4 |
| G719 | 15 | 53.3 | 8.1 | 16.4 | 18 | 78.0 | 13.8 | 26.9 |
| L861 | 15 | 60.0 | 6.0 | 15.2 | 16 | 56.0 | 8.2 | 16.9 |
| Other | 15 | 20.0 | 1.6 | 11.1 | 1 | 100 | – | – |

**Table 5.3 EGFR tyrosine kinase inhibitors and efficacy, according to EGFR status.** OS, overall survival; N, number; PFS, progression-free survival; RR, response rate; TKI, tyrosine kinase inhibitors. Adapted from Wu et al [94]; Yue et al [97]; Ahn et al [98]; Sequist et al [99].

A recent Asiatic study conducted in 308 Taiwanese patients with NSCLC showed that patients with non-LRE deletions had a significantly lower response rate and shorter progression-free survival than individuals with a classical *EGFR* exon 19 deletion [105].

Exon 20 insertion mutations usually occur in amino acids of the N-lobe of *EGFR* encompassing residues G762 and C775 and are typically located after the C-helix of the tyrosine kinase domain of *EGFR* [94,106]. This region is important in orienting the kinase into a state that controls adenosine triphosphate (ATP) and in EGFR-TKI binding. In preclinical models, exon 20 insertions exhibited resistance to gefitinib and erlotinib, similarly to another exon 20 mutation, the T790M mutation, classically associated with EGFR-TKI acquired resistance [107,108]. In a recently published review, Yasuda et al identified 122 patients with exon 20 *EGFR* mutations with a minority of them (only 20 patients) treated with an EGFR-TKI [109]. In this small population, the response rate was 5%, indicating that reversible EGFR-TKIs are modestly effective in such patients. In our prospective study of gefitinib in patients with NSCLC with *EGFR* amplification [110], no response was observed in the four patients harboring exon 20 *EGFR* mutations. Finally, recent data with afatinib showed that even this irreversible EGFR inhibitor is not effective in the presence of exon 20 insertions [96]. Overall, available data show that *EGFR* exon 20 insertions confer de-novo resistance to gefitinib, erlotinib, or afatinib and patients harboring such mutations are not candidates for a front-line treatment with EGFR-TKIs.

### T790M de novo

The *EGFR* mutation T790M is localized at codon 790 on exon 20 and results in the change of threonine to methionine, thus causing steric hindrance to EGFR-TKIs in crystal analysis or increased affinity for ATP. Although the T790M mutation is generally considered as an acquired event, occurring in approximately 50% of patients with acquired resistance to EGFR-TKIs, during the last few years it has become clear that the mutation may be present within tumors before EGFR-TKI treatment. Initial studies using low-sensitivity methods for *EGFR* mutation detection showed that such an event occurs in approximately 1–3% of cases [50,70,111,112]. One prospective study reported one patient with a T790M mutation, detected in combination with an L858R mutation using direct sequencing, among tumor samples from 98 screened patients [70]. However, direct sequencing might underestimate the prevalence of T790M. Inukai et al analyzed the mutation profiles among samples from 280 patients with NSCLC, 185 of which (66%) were not treated with EGFR-TKIs. Direct sequencing revealed the T790M mutation in 0.4% of patients, while mutant-enriched polymerase chain reaction (PCR) assay detected the mutation in 3.6% [112]. In the IPASS study, T790M was found in 11 of 437 (2.5%) tested samples using PCR analysis [50]. More recently, new high sensitivity techniques allowed the detection of T790M mutation in up to 30–40% of patients also harboring classical *EGFR* mutations. Using PCR, Maheswaran et al found low pretreatment levels of T790M in 38% of patients with *EGFR*-mutated NSCLC [111]. Moreover, progression-free survival following EGFR-TKI therapy was significantly shorter among patients with pretreatment T790M (7.7 months) than in those without it (16.5 months; $P<0.001$). Rosell et al tested 129 NSCLC tumor samples from EGFR-TKI naïve patients using the highly specific TaqMan assay [113]. The T790M was detected in 35% of patients and, on multivariate analysis, was independently and significantly associated with a shorter progression-free survival. The higher frequencies of T790M mutations detected in these last two analyses (35–38%) may have resulted from the use of PCR assays with enhanced sensitivity.

Initial studies suggested that presence of the T790M mutation in EGFR-TKI naïve patients with NSCLC predicted poor outcome to TKI treatment [111,113,114]. A retrospective analysis of three studies with afatinib showed that the drug was modestly effective in patients with the T790M mutation [96]. In the Yang et al study, T790M mutations were detected in 1.6% of cases. In such patients afatinib produced a response rate of 14.3% with a median progression-free survival of only 2.9 months and a median survival of 14.9 months [96]. Conversely, the EURTAC trial, a randomized phase III trial comparing erlotinib versus chemotherapy as first-line therapy in patients with classical *EGFR* mutations, showed that individuals harboring both a classical *EGFR* mutation and the T790M mutation had the longest progression-free survival outcome when treated with erlotinib and survival was longer in the T790M positive population irrespective of the therapy, suggesting that T790M is a positive prognostic factor [115], as illustrated in Figure 5.6.

Overall, these data indicate that the method for detecting T790M mutation is critical for deciding whether or not a patient is suitable for front-line therapy with EGFR-TKIs. When the T790M is detected using a low-sensitivity method, this implies that the mutation is present in the majority of tumor clones and, therefore, the patient may be resistant to gefitinib, erlotinib, or afatinib and may be a candidate for standard chemotherapy. When the T790M mutation is detected using high-sensitivity methods, this suggests that the mutation is present in minor clones and will probably not influence the sensitivity to EGFR-TKIs.

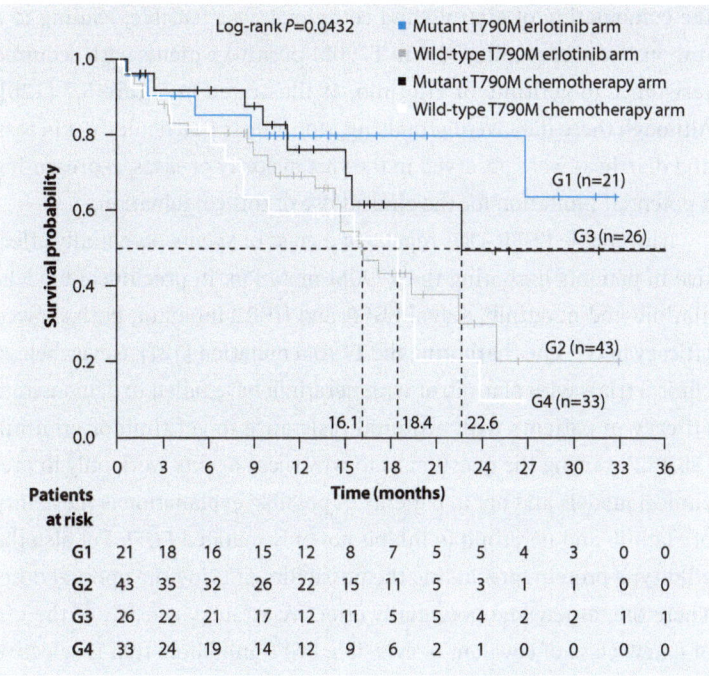

**Figure 5.6 Overall survival by treatment arm and T790M in the EURTAC trial.** Overall survival was not reached for patients with mutant T790M in the erlotinib arm (blue line), 16.1 months for patients with wild-type T790M in the erlotinib arm (grey line), 22.6 months for patients with mutant T790M in the chemotherapy arm (black line), and 18.4 months for patients with wild-type T790M in the chemotherapy arm (white line). Reproduced with permission from © Rosell et al [115].

## *EGFR* mutations and acquired resistance to EGFR tyrosine kinase inhibitors

In approximately half of cases, acquired resistance is caused by the selection of the secondary T790M mutation in *EGFR* (see Figure 5.2 for illustration of the mechanism of action of TKIs in T790M mutations) [114,116,117]. Other secondary point mutations causing EGFR-TKI resistance [118,119] include the replacement of aspartic acid with tyrosine at position 761 (D761Y) and a threonine-to-alanine switch at position 854 (T854A). Treatment of patients with T790M-driven acquired resistance represents a relevant clinical problem. At the present time, standard chemotherapy, including platinum if not previously used, represents the best option available. Nevertheless, new and more effective strategies are currently under investigation. In 2011, Janjigian et al showed that the combination of afatinib and cetuximab was feasible, leading to a response rate exceeding 30% in T790M-positive patients with acquired resistance to gefitinib or erlotinib, as illustrated in Figure 5.7 [120]. Although these data were promising, side effects (particularly skin rash and diarrhea) were observed in the vast majority of cases, representing a potential limitation for the clinical use of this combination.

Irreversible EGFR-TKIs represent a class of agents potentially effective in patients harboring the T790M mutation. In preclinical models, afatinib and neratinib, a dual EGFR and HER2 inhibitor, both showed efficacy in cell lines harboring the T790M mutation [121]. Nevertheless, clinical trials with afatinib or with neratinib have failed to demonstrate efficacy in patients with acquired resistance to gefitinib or erlotinib [58,122], raising the question as to why these agents work only in preclinical models and not in patients. A possible explanation is the ability of afatinib and neratinib to inhibit not only mutated *EGFR* but also the wild-type protein, precluding the possibility of using the optimal dose. Therefore, a new and potentially effective strategy consists of the use of a new class of covalent irreversible EGFR inhibitors that is selective for the mutated form. Several agents are currently under investigation, with very promising results reported with CO-1686 and with AZD 9291 [99,123]. CO-1686, an oral covalent TKI, has been investigated in a phase I/II study [99] enrolling T790M-mutated patients pretreated with

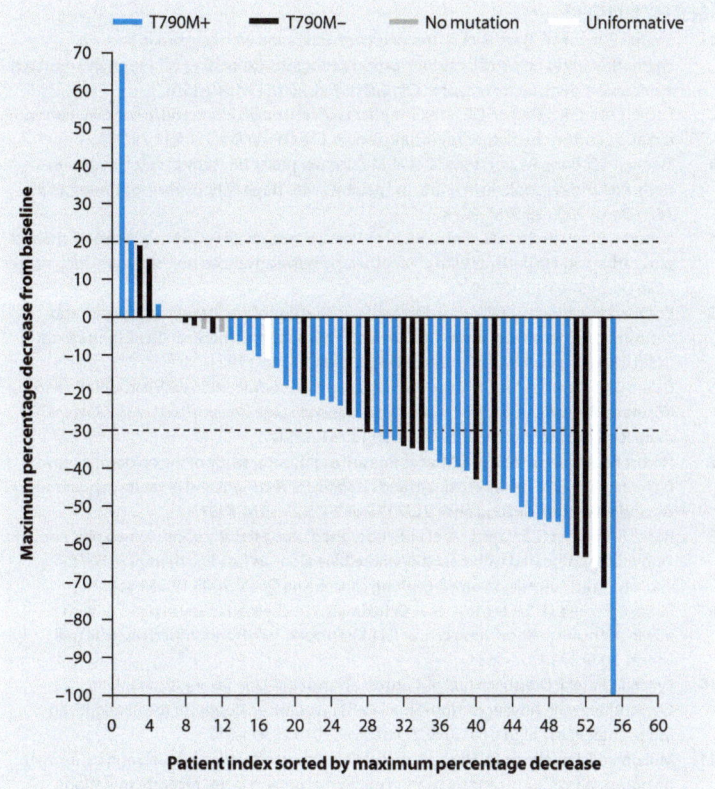

**Figure 5.7 Response to cetuximab–afatinib therapy in a phase I–II trial.** Reproduced with permission from © Janjigian et al [120].

first-generation TKIs. Preliminary results suggested activity and satisfactory tolerability, with the absence of typical adverse events derived from *EGFR* inhibition. AZD 9291 is a potent oral, irreversible inhibitor of *EGFR* that targets EGFR-TKI-sensitizing and resistance mutations. A phase I study showed that this agent is effective in the presence of the T790M mutation even at the lowest used dose, with a very favorable toxicity profile [123].

# References

1   Steiner P, Joynes C, Bassi R, et al. Tumor growth inhibition with cetuximab and chemotherapy in non-small cell lung cancer xenografts expressing wild-type and mutated epidermal growth factor receptor. *Clin Cancer Res.* 2007;13:1540-1551.

2   Raben D, Helfrich B, Chan DC, et al. The effects of cetuximab alone and in combination with radiation and/or chemotherapy in lung cancer. *Clin Cancer Res.* 2005;11:795-805.

3   Thienelt CD, Bunn PA Jr., Hanna N, et al. Multicenter phase I/II study of cetuximab with paclitaxel and carboplatin in untreated patients with stage IV non-small-cell lung cancer. *J Clin Oncol.* 2005;23:8786-9873.

4   Robert F, Blumenschein G, Herbst RS, et al. Phase I/IIa study of cetuximab with gemcitabine plus carboplatin in patients with chemotherapy-naive advanced non-small-cell lung cancer. *J Clin Oncol.* 2005;23:9089-9096.

5   Borghaei H, Langer CJ, Millenson M, et al. Phase II study of paclitaxel, carboplatin, and cetuximab as first line treatment, for patients with advanced non-small cell lung cancer (NSCLC): results of OPN-017. *J Thorac Oncol.* 2008;3:1286-1292.

6   Belani CP, Schreeder MT, Steis RG, et al. Cetuximab in combination with carboplatin and docetaxel for patients with metastatic or advanced-stage nonsmall cell lung cancer: a multicenter phase 2 study. *Cancer.* 2008;113:2512-2517.

7   Herbst RS, Arquette M, Shin DM, et al. Phase II multicenter study of the epidermal growth factor receptor antibody cetuximab and cisplatin for recurrent and refractory squamous cell carcinoma of the head and neck. *J Clin Oncol.* 2005;23:5578-5587.

8   Rosell R, Robinet G, Szczesna A, et al. Randomized phase II study of cetuximab plus cisplatin/vinorelbine compared with cisplatin/vinorelbine alone as first-line therapy in EGFR-expressing advanced non-small-cell lung cancer. *Ann Oncol.* 2008;19:362-369.

9   Pirker R, Pereira JR, Szczesna A, et al. Cetuximab plus chemotherapy in patients with advanced non-small-cell lung cancer (FLEX): an open-label randomised phase III trial. *Lancet.* 2009;373:1525-1531.

10  Lynch TJ, Patel T, Dreisbach L, et al. Cetuximab and First-Line Taxane/Carboplatin Chemotherapy in Advanced Non–Small-Cell Lung Cancer: Results of the Randomized Multicenter Phase III Trial BMS099. *J Clin Oncol.* 2010;28:911-917.

11  Mukohara T, Engelman JA, Hanna NH, et al. Differential effects of gefitinib and cetuximab on non-small-cell lung cancers bearing epidermal growth factor receptor mutations. *J Natl Cancer Inst.* 2005;97:1185-1194.

12  Cappuzzo F, Finocchiaro G, Rossi E, et al. EGFR FISH assay predicts for response to cetuximab in chemotherapy refractory colorectal cancer patients. *Ann Oncol.* 2008;19:717-723.

13  Cappuzzo F, Varella-Garcia M, Finocchiaro G, et al. Primary resistance to cetuximab therapy in EGFR FISH-positive colorectal cancer patients. *B J Cancer.*2008;99:83-89.

14  Herbst RS, Kelly K, Chansky K, et al. Phase II Selection Design Trial of Concurrent Chemotherapy and Cetuximab Versus Chemotherapy Followed by Cetuximab in Advanced-Stage Non–Small-Cell Lung Cancer: Southwest Oncology Group Study S0342. *J Clin Oncol.* 2010;28:4747-4754.

15  Hirsch FR, Herbst RS, Olsen C, et al. Increased EGFR gene copy number detected by fluorescent in situ hybridization predicts outcome in non-small-cell lung cancer patients treated with cetuximab and chemotherapy. *J Clin Oncol.* 2008;26:3351-3357.

16  Khambata-Ford S, Harbison CT, Hart LL, et al. Analysis of potential predictive markers of cetuximab benefit in BMS099, a phase III study of cetuximab and first-line taxane/carboplatin in advanced non-small-cell lung cancer. *J Clin Oncol.* 2010;28:918-927.

17  Karapetis CS, Khambata-Ford S, Jonker DJ, et al. K-ras mutations and benefit from cetuximab in advanced colorectal cancer. *N Engl J Med.* 2008; 359:1757-1765.

18  Pirker R, Pereira JR, von Pawel J, et al. EGFR expression as a predictor of survival for first-line chemotherapy plus cetuximab in patients with advanced non-small-cell lung cancer: analysis of data from the phase 3 FLEX study. *Lancet Oncol.* 2012;13:33-42.

19  First-line Treatment of Participants With Stage IV Squamous Non-Small Cell Lung Cancer With Necitumumab and Gemcitabine-Cisplatin (SQUIRE). ClinicalTrials.gov. www.clinicaltrials.gov/ct2/show/study/NCT00981058. Updated November 16, 2013. Accessed May 27, 2014.

20  Lilly Announces Phase III Necitumumab Study Meets Primary Endpoint of Overall Survival. Lilly. investor.lilly.com/releasedetail.cfm?ReleaseID=784772. Published August 13, 2013. Accessed May 27, 2014.

21  Necitumumab Shows No Benefit in Treating Advanced Non-Squamous Non-Small Cell Lung Cancer: Presented at WCLC. FirstWordPharma. www.firstwordpharma.com/node/1151362?tsid=6#axzz2yTQb9CYR. Published October 13, 2013. Accessed May 27, 2014.

22  Bunn PA Jr, Franklin W. Epidermal growth factor receptor expression, signal pathway, and inhibitors in non-small cell lung cancer. *Semin Oncol*. 2002;29(suppl 14):38-44.

23  Herbst RS, Maddox AM, Rothenberg ML, et al. Selective oral epidermal growth factor receptor tyrosine kinase inhibitor ZD1839 is generally well tolerated and has activity in non-small cell lung cancer and other solid tumors: results of a phase I trial. *J Clin Oncol*. 2002;20:3815-3825.

24  Hidalgo M, Siu LL, Nemunaitis J, et al. Phase I and pharmacologic study of OSI-774, an epidermal growth factor receptor tyrosine kinase inhibitor, in patients with advanced solid malignancies. *J Clin Oncol*. 2001;19:3267-3279.

25  Fukuoka M, Yano S, Giaccone G, et al. Multi-institutional randomized phase II trial of gefitinib for previously treated patients with advanced non-small-cell lung cancer. *J Clin Oncol*. 2003;21:2237-2246.

26  Kris MG, Natale RB, Herbst RS, et al. Efficacy of gefitinib, an inhibitor of the epidermal growth factor receptor tyrosine kinase, in symptomatic patients with non-small cell lung cancer: a randomized trial. *JAMA*. 2003;290:2149-2158.

27  Perez-Soler R, Chachoua A, Huberman M, et al. Final results of a phase II study of erlotinib (Tarceva) monotherapy in patients with advanced nonsmall cell lung cancer following failure of platinum based chemotherapy. *Lung Cancer*. 2003;41(suppl2):S246.

28  Thatcher N, Chang A, Parikh P, et al. Gefitinib plus best supportive care in previously treated patients with refractory advanced non-small-cell lung cancer: results from a randomised, placebo-controlled, multicentre study (Iressa Survival Evaluation in Lung Cancer). *Lancet*. 2005;366:1527-1537.

29  Shepherd FA, Rodrigues PJ, Ciuleanu T, et al. Erlotinib in previously treated non-small-cell lung cancer. *N Engl J Med*. 2005;353:123-132.

30  Maruyama R, Nishiwaki Y, Tamura T, et al. Phase III study, V-15-32, of gefitinib versus docetaxel in previously treated Japanese patients with non-small-cell lung cancer. *J Clin Oncol*. 2008;26:4244-4252.

31  Lee DH, Park K, Kim JH, et al. Randomized Phase III trial of gefitinib versus docetaxel in non-small cell lung cancer patients who have previously received platinum-based chemotherapy. *Clin Cancer Res*. 2010;16:1307-1314.

32  Shepherd FA, Douillard J, Fukuoka M, et al. Comparison of gefitinib and docetaxel in patients with pretreated advanced non-small cell lung cancer (NSCLC): Meta-analysis from four clinical trials. *J Clin Oncol*. 2009;27:15(suppl):8011a.

33  Cufer T, Vrdoljak E, Gaafar R, et al. Phase II, open-label, randomized study (SIGN) of single-agent gefitinib (IRESSA) or docetaxel as second-line therapy in patients with advanced (stage IIIb or IV) non-small-cell lung cancer. *Anticancer Drugs*. 2006;17:401-409.

34  Garassino MC, Martelli O, Broggini M, et al. Erlotinib versus docetaxel as second-line treatment of patients with advanced non-small-cell lung cancer and wild-type EGFR tumours (TAILOR): a randomised controlled trial. *Lancet Oncol*. 2013;14:981-988.

35  Okano Y, Ando M, Asami K, et al. Randomized phase III trial of erlotinib (E) versus docetaxel (D) as second- or third-line therapy in patients with advanced non-small cell lung cancer (NSCLC) who have wild-type or mutant epidermal growth factor receptor (EGFR): Docetaxel and Erlotinib Lung Cancer Trial (DELTA). *J Clin Oncol*. 2013;31(suppl):8006a.

**36**    Lee CK, Brown C, Gralla RJ, et al. Impact of EGFR inhibitor in non-small cell lung cancer on progression-free and overall survival: a meta-analysis. *J Natl Cancer Inst.* 2013;105:595-605.

**37**    Herbst RS, Prager D, Hermann R, et al. TRIBUTE: a phase III trial of erlotinib hydrochloride (OSI-774) combined with carboplatin and paclitaxel chemotherapy in advanced non-small-cell lung cancer. *J Clin Oncol.* 2005;23:5892-5899.

**38**    Giaccone G, Herbst RS, Manegold C, et al. Gefitinib in combination with gemcitabine and cisplatin in advanced non-small-cell lung cancer: a phase III trial--INTACT 1. *J Clin Oncol.* 2004;22:777-784.

**39**    Herbst RS, Giaccone G, Schiller JH, et al. Gefitinib in combination with paclitaxel and carboplatin in advanced non-small-cell lung cancer: a phase III trial--INTACT 2. *J Clin Oncol.* 2004;22:785-794.

**40**    Gatzemeier U, Pluzanska A, Szczesna A, et al. Phase III study of erlotinib in combination with cisplatin and gemcitabine in advanced non-small-cell lung cancer: the Tarceva Lung Cancer Investigation Trial. *J Clin Oncol.* 2007;25:1545-1552.

**41**    Akerley W, Boucher KM, Bentz JS, et al. A phase II study of erlotinib as initial treatment for patients with stage IIIB-IV non-small cell lung cancer. *J Thorac Oncol.* 2009;4:214-219.

**42**    Giaccone G, Gallegos Ruiz M, Le Chevalier T, et al. Erlotinib for frontline treatment of advanced non-small cell lung cancer: a phase II study. *Clin Cancer Res.* 2006;12:6049-6055.

**43**    Niho S, Kubota K, Goto K, et al. First-line single agent treatment with gefitinib in patients with advanced non-small-cell lung cancer: a phase II study. *J Clin Oncol.* 2006;24:64-69.

**44**    Hesketh PJ, Chansky K, Wozniak AJ, et al. Southwest Oncology Group phase II trial (S0341) of erlotinib (OSI-774) in patients with advanced non-small cell lung cancer and a performance status of 2. *J Thorac Oncol.* 2008;3:1026-1031.

**45**    Govindan R, Natale R, Wade J, et al. Efficacy and safety of gefitinib in chemonaive patients with advanced non-small cell lung cancer treated in an Expanded Access Program. *Lung Cancer.* 2006;53:331-337.

**46**    Jackman DM, Yeap BY, Sequist LV, et al. Exon 19 deletion mutations of epidermal growth factor receptor are associated with prolonged survival in non-small cell lung cancer patients treated with gefitinib or erlotinib. *Clin Cancer Res.* 2006;12:3908-3914.

**47**    Gridelli C, Ciardiello F, Gallo C, et al. First-line erlotinib followed by second-line cisplatin-gemcitabine chemotherapy in advanced non-small-cell lung cancer: the TORCH randomized trial. *J Clin Oncol.* 2012;30:3002-3011.

**48**    Lee SM, Khan I, Upadhyay S, et al. First-line erlotinib in patients with advanced non-small-cell lung cancer unsuitable for chemotherapy (TOPICAL): a double-blind, placebo-controlled, phase 3 trial. *Lancet Oncol.* 2012;13:1161-1170.

**49**    Crinò L, Cappuzzo F, Zatloukal P, et al. Gefitinib versus vinorelbine in chemotherapy-naive elderly patients with advanced non-small-cell lung cancer (INVITE): a randomized, phase II study. *J Clin Oncol.* 2008;26:4253-4260.

**50**    Fukuoka M, Wu YL, Thongprasert S, et al. Biomarker analyses and final overall survival results from a phase III, randomized, open-label, first-line study of gefitinib versus carboplatin/paclitaxel in clinically selected patients with advanced non-small-cell lung cancer in Asia (IPASS). *J Clin Oncol.* 2011;29:2866-2874.

**51**    Johnson BE, Kabbinavar F, Fehrenbacher L, et al. ATLAS: randomized, double-blind, placebo-controlled, phase IIIB trial comparing bevacizumab therapy with or without erlotinib, after completion of chemotherapy, with bevacizumab for first-line treatment of advanced non-small-cell lung cancer. *J Clin Oncol.* 2013;31:3926-3934.

**52**    Takeda K, Hida T, Sato T, et al. Randomized phase III trial of platinum-doublet chemotherapy followed by gefitinib compared with continued platinum-doublet chemotherapy in Japanese patients with advanced non-small-cell lung cancer: results of a west Japan thoracic oncology group trial (WJTOG0203). *J Clin Oncol.* 2010;28:753-760.

**53** Kelly K, Chansky K, Gaspar LE, et al. Phase III trial of maintenance Gefitinib or placebo after concurrent chemoradiotherapy and docetaxel consolidation in inoperable stage III non-small-cell lung cancer: SWOG S0023. *J Clin Oncol.* 2008;26:2450-2456.

**54** Zhang L, Ma S, Song X, et al. Gefitinib versus placebo as maintenance therapy in patients with locally advanced or metastatic non-small-cell lung cancer (INFORM; C-TONG 0804): a multicentre, double-blind randomised phase 3 trial. *Lancet Oncol.* 2012;13:466-475.

**55** Li D, Ambrogio L, Shimamura T, et al. BIBW2992, an irreversible EGFR/HER2 inhibitor highly effective in preclinical lung cancer models. *Oncogene.* 2008;27:4702-4711.

**56** Nelson V, Ziehr J, Agulnik M, Johnson M. Afatinib: emerging next-generation tyrosine kinase inhibitor for NSCLC. *Onco Targets Ther.* 2013;6:135-143.

**57** Yap TA, Vidal L, Adam J, et al. Phase I trial of the irreversible ErbB1 (EGFR) and ErbB2 (HER2) kinase inhibitor BIBW 2992 in patients with advanced solid tumours. *J Clin Oncol.* 2010;28:3965-7392.

**58** Miller VA, Hirsh V, Cadranel J, et al. Afatinib versus placebo for patients with advanced, metastatic non- small-cell lung cancer after failure of erlotinib, gefitinib, or both, and one or two lines of chemotherapy (LUX- Lung 1): a phase 2b/3 randomised trial. *Lancet Oncol.* 2012;13:528-538.

**59** Han JY, Park K, Kim SW, et al. First-SIGNAL: first-line single-agent IRESSA versus gemcitabine and cisplatin trial in never-smokers with adenocarcinoma of the lung. *J Clin Oncol.* 2012;30:1122-1128.

**60** Mok TS, Wu YL, Thongprasert S, et al. Gefitinib or carboplatin-paclitaxel in pulmonary adenocarcinoma. *N Engl J Med.* 2009;361:947-957.

**61** Mitsudomi T, Morita S, Yatabe Y, et al. Gefitinib versus cisplatin plus docetaxel in patients with non-small cell lung cancer harbouring mutations of the epidermal growth factor receptor (WJTOG3405): An open label, randomised phase 3 trial. *Lancet Oncol.* 2010;11:121-128.

**62** Maemondo M, Inoue A, Kobayashi K, et al. Gefitinib or chemotherapy for non–small-cell lung cancer with mutated EGFR. *N Engl J Med.* 2010;362:2380-2388.

**63** Zhou C, Wu YL, Chen G, et al. Erlotinib versus chemotherapy as first-line treatment for patients with advanced EGFR mutation-positive non-small cell lung cancer (OPTIMAL, CTONG-0802): A multicentre, open-label, randomised, phase 3 study. *Lancet Oncol.* 2011;12:735-742.

**64** Rosell R, Carcereny E, Gervais R, et al. Erlotinib versus standard chemotherapy as first-line treatment for European patients with advanced EGFR mutation-positive non-small-cell lung cancer (EURTAC): A multicentre, open-label, randomised phase 3 trial. *Lancet Oncol.* 2012;13:239-246.

**65** Sequist LV, Yang JC, Yamamoto N, et al. Phase III study of afatinib or cisplatin plus pemetrexed in patients with metastatic lung adenocarcinoma with EGFR mutations. *J Clin Oncol.* 2012;31:3327-3334.

**66** Wu YL, Zhou C, Hu CP, et al. Afatinib versus cisplatin plus gemcitabine for first-line treatment of Asian patients with advanced non-small-cell lung cancer harbouring EGFR mutations (LUX-Lung 6): an open-label, randomised phase 3 trial. *Lancet Oncol.* 2014; 15:213-222.

**67** Asahina H, Yamazaki K, Kinoshita I, et al. A phase II trial of gefitinib as first-line therapy for advanced non-small-cell lung cancer with epidermal growth factor receptor mutations. *Br J Cancer.* 2006;95:998-1004.

**68** Inoue A, Suzuki T, Fukuhara T, et al. Prospective phase II study of gefitinib for chemotherapy naive patients with advanced non-small-cell lung cancer with epidermal growth factor receptor gene mutations. *J Clin Oncol.* 2006;24:3340-3346.

**69** Yang C, Yu C, Shih J, et al. Specific EGFR mutations predict treatment outcome of stage IIIB/IV patients with chemotherapy-naive non-small cell lung cancer receiving first-line gefitinib monotherapy. *J Clin Oncol.* 2008;26:2745-2753.

**70** Sequist LV, Martins RG, Spigel D, et al. First-line gefitinib in patients with advanced non-small-cell lung cancer harboring somatic EGFR mutations. *J Clin Oncol.* 2008;26:2442-2449.

71    Inoue A, Kobayashi K, Usui K, et al. First-line gefitinib for patients with advanced non-small-cell lung cancer harboring epidermal growth factor receptor mutations without indication for chemotherapy. *J Clin Oncol*. 2009;27:1394-1400.

72    Sutani A, Nagai Y, Udagawa K, et al. Gefitinib for non-small-cell lung cancer patients with epidermal growth factor receptor gene mutations screened by peptide nucleic acid-locked nucleic acid PCR clamp. *Br J Cancer*. 2006;95:1483-1489.

73    Yoshida K, Yatabe Y, Park JY, et al. Prospective validation of prediction of gefitinib sensitivity by epidermal growth factor receptor gene mutation in patients with non-small cell lung cancer. *J Thorac Oncol*. 2007;2:22-28.

74    Sunaga N, Tomizawa Y, Yanagitani N, et al. Phase II prospective study of the efficacy of gefitinib for the treatment of stage III/IV non-small cell lung cancer with EGFR mutations, irrespective of previous chemotherapy. *Lung Cancer*. 2007;56:383-389.

75    Tamura K, Okamoto I, Kashii T, et al. Multicentre prospective phase II trial of gefitinib for advanced non-small cell lung cancer with epidermal growth factor receptor mutations: results of the West Japan Thoracic Oncology Group trial (WJTOG0403). *Br J Cancer*. 2008;98:907-914.

76    Sugio K, Uramoto H, Onitsuka T, et al. Prospective phase II study of gefitinib in non-small cell lung cancer with epidermal growth factor receptor mutations. *Lung Cancer*. 2009;64:314-318.

77    Rosell R, Moran T, Queralt C, et al. Screening for epidermal growth factor receptor mutations in lung cancer. *N Engl J Med*. 2009;361:958-967.

78    Yang JC, Shih JY, Su WC, et al. Afatinib for patients with lung adenocarcinoma and epidermal growth factor receptor mutations (LUX-Lung 2): A phase 2 trial. *Lancet Oncol*. 2012;13:539-548.

79    Yang JC-H, Schuler M, Yamamoto N, et al; on behalf of LUX-Lung 3 investigators. LUX-Lung 3: a randomized, open-label, Phase III study of afatinib vs cisplatin/pemetrexed as 1st-line treatment for patients with advanced adenocarcinoma of the lung harboring EGFR-activating mutations. Slides presented at: 2012 ASCO Annual Meeting; June 1-June 5, 2013; Chicago, IL. Abstract LBA7500.

80    Yang JC, Hirsh V, Schuler M, et al. Symptom Control and Quality of Life in LUX-Lung 3: A Phase III Study of Afatinib or Cisplatin/Pemetrexed in Patients With Advanced Lung Adenocarcinoma With EGFR Mutations. *J Clin Oncol*. 2013;31:3342-3350.

81    Engelman JA, Zejnullahu K, Gale CM, et al. PF00299804, an irreversible pan-ERBB inhibitor, is effective in lung cancer models with EGFR and ERBB2 mutations that are resistant to gefitinib. *Cancer Res*. 2007;67:11924-11932.

82    Janne PA, Schellens JH, Engleman JA, et al. Preliminary activity and safety results from a phase I clinical trial of PF-00299804, an irreversible pan-HER inhibitor, in patients (pts) with NSCLC. *J Clin Oncol*. 2008;26(15 Suppl);8027.

83    Campbell A, Reckamp KL, Camidge DR, et al. PF-00299804 (PF299) patient-reported outcomes and efficacy in adenocarcinoma and non adeno non-small cell lung cancer: a phase 2 trial in advanced NSCLC after failure of chemotherapy and erlotinib. *J Clin Oncol*. 2010;28(15 suppl):7602.

84    Ramalingam S, Blackhall F, Krzakowski M, et al. Randomized phase II study of dacomitinib (PF-00299804), an irreversible pan-human epidermal growth factor receptor inhibitor, versus erlotinib in patients with advanced non-small-cell lung cancer. *J Clin Oncol*. 2012;30:3337-3344.

85    Boyer M, Janne PA, Mok T, et al. ARCHER: Dacomitinib (D; PF-00299804) versus erlotinib (E) for advanced (adv) non-small cell lung cancer (NSCLC)—A randomized double-blind phase III study. *J Clin Oncol*. 2012;30(suppl):TPS7615a.

86    Pfizer Announces Top-Line Results From Two Phase 3 Trials Of Dacomitinib In Patients With Refractory Advanced Non-Small Cell Lung Cancer. Pfizer. www.pfizer.com/news/press-release/press-release-detail/pfizer_announces_top_line_results_from_two_phase_3_trials_of_dacomitinib_in_patients_with_refractory_advanced_non_small_cell_lung_cancer. Published January 27, 2014. Accessed May 27, 2014.

87    Kris MG, Mok T, Ou SH, et al. First-line dacomitinib (PF-00299804), an irreversible pan-HER tyrosine kinase inhibitor, for patients with EGFR-mutant lung cancers. *J Clin Oncol*. 2012;30(suppl):7602a.

88    Mok T, Nakagawa K, Rosell R, et al. Phase III randomized, open label study (ARCHER 1050) of first-line dacomitinib (D) versus gefitinib (G) for advanced (adv) non-small cell lung cancer (NSCLC) in patients (pts) with epidermal growth factor receptor (*EGFR*) activating mutation(s). *J Clin Oncol*. 2013;31(suppl):TPS8123a.

89    Mitsudomi T, Kosaka T, Endoh H, et al. Mutations of the epidermal growth factor receptor gene predict prolonged survival after gefitinib treatment in patients with non-small-cell lung cancer with postoperative recurrence. *J Clin Oncol*. 2005;23:2513-2520.

90    Riely GJ, Pao W, Pham D, et al. Clinical course of patients with non-small cell lung cancer and epidermal growth factor receptor exon 19 and exon 21 mutations treated with gefitinib or erlotinib. *Clin Cancer Res*. 2006;12:839-844.

91    Jackman DM, Miller VA, Cioffredi LA, et al. Impact of epidermal growth factor receptor and KRAS mutations on clinical outcomes in previously untreated non-small cell lung cancer patients: results of an online tumor registry of clinical trials. *Clin Cancer Res*. 2009;15:5267-5273.

92    Sholl LM, Yeap BY, Iafrate AJ, et al. Lung adenocarcinoma with EGFR amplification has distinct clinicopathologic and molecular features in never-smokers. *Cancer Res*. 2009;69:8341-8348.

93    Carey KD, Garton AJ, Romero MS, et al. Kinetic analysis of epidermal growth factor receptor somatic mutant proteins shows increased sensitivity to the epidermal growth factor receptor tyrosine kinase inhibitor, erlotinib. *Cancer Res*. 2006;66:8163-8171.

94    Mitsudomi T, Yatabe Y. Mutations of the epidermal growth factor receptor gene and related genes as determinants of the epidermal growth factor receptor tyrosine kinase inhibitors sensitivity in lung cancer. *Cancer Sci*. 2007;98:1817-1824.

95    Wu JY, Yu CJ, Chang YC, et al. Effectiveness of tyrosine kinase inhibitors on "uncommon" epidermal growth factor receptor mutations of unknown clinical significance in non-small-cell lung cancer. *Clin Cancer Res*. 2011;17:3812-3821.

96    Yang J C-H, Sequist L, Geater SL, et al. Activity of afatinib in uncommon epidermal growth factor receptor (EGFR) mutations: findings from three trials of afatinib in EGFR mutation positive lung cancer. *J Thor Oncol*. 2013;8(suppl2):S141.

97    Yue D, Xu S, Li Q, et al. A prospective, open-labeled, randomized, multicenter phase II study to evaluate efficacy and safety of erlotinib vs np chemotherapy as adjuvant therapy in post radical operation stage IIIA NSCLC patients with EGFR 19 or 21 exon mutation (EVAN, ML28280, NCT01683175). Poster presented at the 15th World Conference on Lung Cancer; October 27-October 30, 2013; Sydney, Australia.

98    Ahn M-JA, Kim SW, Cho BC, et al. Phase II trial of afatinib as a third-line treatment for Korean patients (pts) with wild-type epidermal growth factor receptor (WTEGFR) stage IIIB/IV lung adenocarcinoma. Presented at the 37th ESMO Congress; September 28-October 2, 2012. Abstract 878.

99    Sequist LV, Soria JC, Gadgeel SM, et al. First-in-human evaluation of CO-1686, an irreversible, selective, and potent tyrosine kinase inhibitor of EGFR T790M. *J Clin Oncol*. 2013;31(suppl):2524a.

100   Ilie MI, Hofman V, Bonnetaud C, et al. Usefullness of tissue microarrays for assessment of protein expression, gene copy number and mutational status of EGFR in lung adenocarcinoma. *Virchows Arch*. 2010;457:483-495.

101   Tsao MS, Sakurada A, Cutz JC, et al. Erlotinib in lung cancer - molecular and clinical predictors of outcome. *N Engl J Med*. 2005;353:133–144.

102   De Pas T, Toffalorio F, Manzotti M, et al. Activity of epidermal growth factor receptor-tyrosine kinase inhibitors in patients with non-small cell lung cancer harboring rare epidermal growth factor receptor mutations. *J Thorac Oncol*. 2011;6:1895-1901.

**103** He M, Capelletti M, Nafa K, et al. EGFR exon 19 insertions: a new family of sensitizing EGFR mutations in lung adenocarcinoma. *Clin Cancer Res.* 2012;18:1790-1797.

**104** Gazdar AF. Activating and resistance mutations of EGFR in non-small-cell lung cancer: role in clinical response to EGFR tyrosine kinase inhibitors. *Oncogene.* 2009;28(Suppl 1):S24-S31.

**105** Chung KP, Wu SG, Wu JY, et al. Clinical outcomes in non-small cell lung cancer harboring different exon 19 deletions in EGFR. *Clin Cancer Res.* 2012;18:3470-3477.

**106** Pao W, Chmielecki J. Rational, biologically based treatment of EGFR-mutant non-small-cell lung cancer. *Nat Rev Cancer.* 2010;10:760-764.

**107** Kobayashi S, Boggon TJ, Dayaram T, et al. EGFR mutation and resistance of non-small-cell lung cancer to gefitinib. *N Engl J Med.* 2005;352:786-792.

**108** Kobayashi S, Ji H, Yuza Y, et al. An alternative inhibitor overcomes resistance caused by a mutation of the epidermal growth factor receptor. *Cancer Res.* 2005;65:7096-7101.

**109** Yasuda H, Kobayashi S, Costa DB, et al. EGFR exon 20 insertion mutations in non-small-cell lung cancer: preclinical data and clinical implications. *Lancet Oncol.* 2012;13:e23-e31.

**110** Cappuzzo F, Ligorio C, Jänne PA, et al. Prospective study of gefitinib in epidermal growth factor receptor fluorescence in situ hybridization-positive/phospho-Akt-positive or never smoker patients with advanced non-small-cell lung cancer: the ONCOBELL trial. *J Clin Oncol.* 2007;25:2248-2255.

**111** Maheswaran S, Sequist LV, Nagrath S, et al. Detection of mutations in EGFR in circulating lung-cancer cells. *N Engl J Med.* 2008;359:366-377.

**112** Inukai M, Toyooka S, Ito S, et al. Presence of epidermal growth factor receptor gene T790M mutation as a minor clone in non-small cell lung cancer. *Cancer Res.* 2006;66:7854-7858.

**113** Rosell R, Molina MA, Costa C, et al. Pretreatment EGFR T790M mutation and BRCA1 mRNA expression in erlotinib-treated advanced non-small-cell lung cancer patients with EGFR mutations. *Clin Cancer Res.* 2011;17:1160-1168.

**114** Su KY, Chen HY, Li KC, et al. Pretreatment Epidermal Growth Factor Receptor (EGFR) T790M mutation predicts shorter EGFR tyrosine kinase inhibitor response duration in patients with non-small-cell lung cancer. *J Clin Oncol.* 2012;30:433-440.

**115** Rosell R, Molina-Vila MA, Taron M, et al. EGFR compound mutants and survival on erlotinib in non-small cell lung cancer (NSCLC) patients (p) in the EURTAC study. *J Clin Oncol.* 2012;30(suppl):7522a.

**116** Pao W, Miller VA, Politi KA, et al. Acquired resistance of lung adenocarcinomas to gefitinib or erlotinib is associated with a second mutation in the EGFR kinase domain. *PLoS Med.* 2005;2:e73.

**117** Yun CH, Mengwasser KE, Toms AV, et al. The T790M mutation in EGFR kinase causes drug resistance by increasing the affinity for ATP. *Proc Natl Acad Sci U S A.* 2008;105:2070-2075.

**118** Balak MN, Gong Y, Riely GJ, et al. Novel D761Y and common secondary T790M mutations in epidermal growth factor receptor-mutant lung adenocarcinomas with acquired resistance to kinase inhibitors. *Clin Cancer Res.* 2006;12:6494-6501.

**119** Bean J, Riely GJ, Balak M, et al. Acquired resistance to epidermal growth factor receptor kinase inhibitors associated with a novel T854A mutation in a patient with EGFR-mutant lung adenocarcinoma. *Clin Cancer Res.* 2008;14:7519-7525.

**120** Janjigian YY, Groen HJ, Horn L, et al. Activity and tolerability of afatinib (BIBW 2992) and cetuximab in NSCLC patients with acquired resistance to erlotinib or gefitinib. *J Clin Oncol.* 2011;29(suppl):7525a.

**121** Rabindran SK, Discafani CM, Rosfjord EC, et al. Antitumor activity of HKI-272, an orally active, irreversible inhibitor of the HER-2 tyrosine kinase. *Cancer Res.* 2004;64:3958-3965.

**122** Sequist LV, Besse B, Lynch TJ, et al. Neratinib, an irreversible pan-ErbB receptor tyrosine kinase inhibitor: results of a phase II trial in patients with advanced non-small-cell lung cancer. *J Clin Oncol.* 2010;28:3076-3083.

**123** Ranson M, Pao W, Kim DW, et al. Preliminary results from a Phase I study with AZD9291: An irreversible inhibitor of epidermal growth factor receptor (EGFR) activating and resistance mutations in non-small-cell lung cancer (NSCLC). *Eur J Cancer.* 2013;49 (suppl);LBA33.

# Chapter 6

# Conclusions

Cancer treatment is moving towards individualized therapy and biomarker analysis is becoming the most important element for basing treatment decisions. In patients with non-small cell lung cancer (NSCLC) it is now mandatory to evaluate *epidermal growth factor receptor (EGFR)* mutation status before treatment choice and EGFR tyrosine kinase inhibitors (TKIs) are the optimal option in the patients harboring activating *EGFR* mutations. Although *EGFR* assessment is sometimes difficult in clinical practice for several reasons, including availability of sufficient tumor tissue or facilities, every effort should be made to assess *EGFR* status in patients with NSCLC. Unfortunately, even in individuals with *EGFR* mutations, no patient with metastatic disease can obtain a definitive cure. In the near future, the routine care for patients with NSCLC is likely to involve a molecular 'portrait' that will provide information about the prognosis and the best targeted therapy directed at the specific mutation. *EGFR*-mutated NSCLC is likely to be treated increasingly as a chronic illness owing to its relatively good prognosis. This will require a paradigm shift whereby the use of palliative chemotherapy is replaced by long-term treatment and monitoring. A second generation of molecular targeted agents in development for NSCLC is likely to offer important benefits over current EGFR-TKIs, especially in the management of resistant tumors.

© Springer International Publishing Switzerland 2014
F. Cappuzzo, *Guide to Targeted Therapies: EGFR mutations in NSCLC*, DOI 10.1007/978-3-319-03059-3_6